She Does Not Fear the Snow

Bobbie Ann Cole

She Does Not Fear the Snow

Scriptures taken from the Holy Bible, New International Version®, NIV®. Copyright © 1973, 1978, 1984, 2011 by Biblica, Inc.™ Used by permission of Zondervan. All rights reserved worldwide.www.zondervan.com The "NIV" and "New International Version" are trademarks registered in the United States Patent and Trademark Office by Biblica, Inc.™
Print ISBN: 978-0-9917604-2-8
E-book ISBN: 978-0-9917604-3-5

This book is based on the author's experiences. In order to protect privacy, some names and identifying characteristics have been changed or reconstructed.

Cover design: Erin Johnson
Formatting: RikHall.com

To Butch, of course...

'He reached down from on high and took hold of me. He drew me out of deep waters.'
2 Samuel 22:17

'Take a scroll and write on it all the words I have spoken to you concerning Israel, Judah and all the other nations from the time I began speaking to you.'
Jeremiah 36:2

For we did not follow cleverly devised stories when we told you about the coming of our Lord Jesus Christ in power, but we were eyewitnesses of his majesty.
2 Peter 1:16

A proportion of the proceeds of this work will be donated to Alpha International and/or Alpha Canada.

The Alpha Course was founded by Holy Trinity Church Brompton in London and has spread throughout the world, introducing people to who Jesus was and what He stands for.

Alpha invites you to lift the lid on all your nagging questions. Leave no stone unturned. Alpha is your open door.'

http://www.alphacanada.org/

A Note from the Author

This is not a neat story with all the loose ends tied up. It is a true story of a series of miraculous events I lived through.

I do not have a ready explanation for everything that happened but I firmly believe God was leading me, every step of the way.

See the *She Does Not Fear the Snow* Photo Gallery at pics.shedoesnotfearthesnow.com.

Bobbie Ann Cole

Praise for She Does Not Fear the Snow

'Filled with humor, warmth and love, *She Does Not Fear the Snow* is the promise of love after a battle with cancer and the sting of divorce. Bobbie Ann Cole has written an honest, touching memoir which permits the reader to accompany her through a time of healing, self-discovery and faith. Bobbie's transparency makes it hard to put down. A great read for those healing from their own journey. You will find encouragement here.'

Kim de Blecourt, Author of *Until We All Come Home: A Harrowing Journey, a Mother's Courage, a Race to Freedom* (FaithWords, November, 2012)

'*She Does Not Fear the Snow* is much more than Bobbie Cole's testimony about her journey into faith in Jesus Christ. It is an adventure, a tale of endurance, a love story and a thrilling reminder of God's Father Heart towards his people. This remarkable book is a must for anyone who believes that God is uncaring, distant and remote from our everyday lives. Here, in these pages carved from one woman's experience of God's very specific guidance, is the revelation that God watches over each one of us in the most incredible and intimate way.'

Trevor Payne, Senior Pastor, Hope Church, Bromley, England

'This story shows the amazing love and power of God working through relationships to bring healing, especially spiritual healing. God's presence is obvious through the signs and visions given to those who seek the Lord like the author.'

Kathy Bruins, Christian author, speaker and dramatist

'*She Does Not Fear the Snow* will keep you turning the pages until the very last word. This book will inspire you to look for God's voice in everyday events of life. It will cause you to reflect on past experiences and see how God's handled you in the right path. It's a beautiful story full of romance, forgiveness and coming to faith.'

Evangeline Inman, Author of *The Divine Heartmender* and *Extreme Worship for Songwriters*

'Is there more to life than what we see? Bobbie Cole's story, written with both deep insight and humble humour, is a captivating account of what happens when the supernatural envelopes her life's struggles of womanhood, marriage, and faith. This is a must read story of hope and healing, exemplifying that there is a God who lets us find Him when we seek Him.'

Jill Kozak, Creative Arts Director, Smythe Street Cathedral, Fredericton, NB, Canada

'An ordinary woman with Jewish heritage discovers that her talents are God-given, her life does have purpose and there is a Messiah who loves unconditionally. A must-read for the questioner, the wonderer and the broken.'

George Woodward, Director, Israel's Peace Ministries

'I was completely drawn into Bobbie's journey from pain and loss to finding faith as I read her compelling story. She writes with an openness and transparency that speaks directly to the heart, giving us hope that there is One who hears our deepest cry and responds with love beyond all expectation!'

Rita Tsukahira, Co-Director, *Or HaCarmel* Center, Israel

'Once I started reading *She Does Not Fear The Snow* I couldn't put it down. I really enjoy a well written story and that's how this book starts. But beyond a good story there is a powerful message of hope. This story will inspire you, encourage you and entertain you. The truth is overwhelming in a good way.'

Kimanzi Constable, Author, Speaker, Consultant

'In my friendship and role as a pastor to Bobbie and her husband Butch, I have sensed and seen in them the longing for, the pursuit of and the realization of God's destiny for their lives. Bobbie's story greatly encourages us that life is not to be lived or viewed through the lens of chance. Open your heart as you read, and embrace the personal truth that God in His providence will direct our steps and bring us to our destiny.'

Pastor Wayne Flowers, Smythe Street Cathedral, Fredericton, NB, Canada

Acknowledgements

My thanks go, first and foremost, to my husband, Butch, for being there, encouraging me and shouldering the burden of what I couldn't do around the house because I was writing this book.

Thanks also to my family who always have my best interests at heart. I love you all very much.

I have received much help, support, feedback and encouragement from a number of friends during the course of this four-year project. I would like, in particular, to recognise my dear friend, Valerie Letley. She is a woman with whom you can dream what might be and then practically turn that dream into reality.

Valerie scripted, directed and produced the beautiful promo video for this book, which was edited by Jenny Albrecht. You can see this at:

www.shedoesnotfearthesnow.com

I am grateful to Sara Maitland for her feedback on an early version of this book. Also a big 'thank you' to Beth Jusino, my editor, who totally helped me sort out what I thought was the final copy.

I am indebted to Erin Johnson, my dedicated designer.

Finally, thanks go to my endorsers, who were obliged to read my MSS in pdf format, and to my Launch Project Team for their input and energy.

Chapter 1

1.

'These are for my brother, Butch,' my friend, Terry, enthused. She had begun snapping pictures almost as soon as we slid into the row near the back of the crowded auditorium. 'He'd love this.'

Taking pictures inside a church, with a service going on, seemed sacrilegious to me. As a Jew, it was something I would never have done in a synagogue.

As a Jew, I shouldn't be here at all.

Clearly things were different in Christian worship, starting with the unexpected wave of human warmth that hit me in the face as we stepped into this former cinema, located in the basement of a somewhat seedy, Jerusalem shopping mall. The location felt weird. You don't find synagogues in basements. The rule is that nothing, other than the synagogue ceiling, is supposed to come between the Almighty and the worshipper.

Everything else was weird, too. People were on their feet, waving their arms. Pop praise was being sung and played on electric guitars and drums. There were no hymn sheets or prayer books: all the words were flashed up on a screen behind the band. They were in English not Hebrew, even though we were in Israel.

The atmosphere in my home synagogue back in England was nothing like this. It was formal and detached. Most of the service was in Hebrew.

As for the synagogue Terry and I had visited here in Jerusalem on Friday night, well, for all the welcome anyone gave us there, we might have been invisible. In fact, Terry, who loved mystique, had suggested we might actually have been rendered invisible during our time there.

The fact that she had accompanied me then was the *only* reason I was here now, at Sunday evening worship in a Christian church.

The music paused. We were invited to greet those around us. I introduced myself to a German man on my right and an Irish-looking man — with tweeds, jug ears and tight ginger curls — in the row in front.

Another man was making his way toward us, weaving through the people in the back row, immediately behind us. His appearance was shabby. He wore a black raincoat over an ankle-length tunic and sandals on his feet. His beard was ragged, his long, black hair untidy.

Beaming broadly, he shook our hands. It was as if he had been looking out for us, as if we were expected. His surprising air of authority led me to take him for an eccentric elder, even though his appearance didn't seem to fit with this middle-class, Canadian-led congregation.

The music struck up again and I soon forgot him as everyone started singing and praising God. Sweet music was all around me. In one ear, Terry's voice, deep and resonant and full of soul, gave the lie to her Barbie doll topknot and petite frame. In the other was my German neighbour, a hearty baritone.

The singing was stirring. I found myself feeling grateful to be here, grateful for this moment.

Now I noticed the Irish-looking man in the row in front of me. As he praised God, he was giving out what I can only describe as invisible waves of energy. They rose like a vapour to envelop me. Their effect was to fill me with electricity, yet, paradoxically, they also made me relax, like I was leaning back into a warm bath.

I let out a long sigh as the love given out by the congregation overwhelmed me. Tears sprang to my eyes and a lump formed in my throat. I remained very still as the world around me moved.

I wanted more of this balm, more of this acute awareness of love. I put out a hand to connect with the man in front, to touch his shoulder... but withdrew, not daring to go that far.

'*Hineini*,' I whispered.

This is Hebrew for *here I am*, a phrase found over and over in the Bible. God often told his followers *hineini*. Abraham, Jacob and Moses said *hineini* when they responded to His call.

Ahead of this trip, I had been telling God *hineini*. After five years of sickness that included cancer, my marriage had crumpled and my business had failed. I had been living alone for eighteen months, wondering what to do.

Hineini was my plea for a fresh start. I wanted some meaning and purpose.

My friend and fellow traveller, Terry, was also looking for something. We first met when holidaying with our respective kids in Alberta twenty years before. We hit it off straight away, even though we were about as different as any two friends could be. She was small,

I was tallish. She was blond, I was dark. But our differences went way beyond the physical. She was a dreamer, I was a pragmatist. Though she was living just outside Vancouver at the time, she was a country girl from rural New Brunswick, Canada. I was from fast-paced London, England. She was a Christian, I was a Jew.

We both loved the Land of Israel and viewed it as God's home. When I told her of my plans to make Israel the destination of my spiritual quest, she initially called me a 'stinker'. A few days later, she announced she was coming along with me.

At the Western Wall in Jerusalem's Old City, the most holy place in the world for Jews, she had added two notes of her own to the pleas on scraps of paper that flutter in the cracks between the stones. One of them was a prayer given to her by that same brother she had eagerly snapped photos for when we came in. The other was her own message, which, she told me, said, 'I'm your girl'. I thought that sounded pretty much the same as '*hineini*'.

Our search had taken us all over Israel, without any clear idea what it was we were hoping to find. We had seen some stunningly beautiful places but found little evidence of spirituality in the cars and Coca Cola hoardings of this rapidly westernising country.

Now, tonight, something special was happening. And it was happening in a Christian church, of all places.

The music stopped again and everyone sat down. A guest preacher, a pastor from Germany, began to speak. His English was so bad and his accent so thick that I thought him brave to stand up and use it.

His subject matter was stirring, however. He talked to us about healing, about mending divisions, about forgiveness and becoming peacemakers. The idea of becoming a peacemaker appealed to me, though I realised that my first step in that direction would mean forgiving my former husband, which I would find a very hard call. Even though I knew that an unforgiving attitude was keeping me in a sticky place and preventing me from moving on, there did not seem to be very much I could do about it.

As he began his closing prayer, he broke off to say, 'I feel that there is a woman here tonight who wants to become a child. May she become one.'

I was pretty sure he was getting mixed up with his verbs and using the German verb *bekommen*, which means 'to get'. He thought he was reassuring a woman who wanted to get pregnant. But it spoke to me and seemed like a right mistake: I was the woman who wanted to become a child. If only someone would take me by the hand and lead me.

All too soon, it seemed, people were getting to their feet and putting on their coats. (It can be cold in Jerusalem in March. Ten days before, when we arrived, it was snowing.)

I had not wanted to come and now I didn't want to leave. I remained in my seat, with the power I had absorbed still flowing through me. The service had closed with an invitation to go up to the 24/7 Prayer Tower. I hoped with all my heart that Terry would be willing to go there with me.

She didn't seem in any hurry to get going. As the place emptied, she continued sitting quietly beside me, reviewing the photographs on her camera's digital display. Like me, she seemed bewildered. In fact, she was frowning.

I was about to ask her why when the Irish-looking man pulled up his collar. He was poised to brave the cold outside. I had to tell him. Having no idea what I was going to say, I watched my hand reach out to touch his elbow.

'I could feel your faith, washing over me,' I said.

To my relief, he didn't smirk.

'It was special,' he agreed. 'There were angels here tonight.' His accent was North American, not Irish at all.

He turned towards the exit. 'God bless you.'

'God bless you,' I replied. The unfamiliar words hung like pebbles in my mouth.

Terry looked up, her eyes like saucers. 'There *were* angels here tonight, Bobbie. They're in my camera!'

She held it out for me to take.

I studied the digital display. The first picture was of a military tank we saw in the Jaffa Road, immediately before we came in. There was nothing remarkable about it, beyond the presence of a tank in a downtown shopping street.

The next picture, taken here, where we now sat, was something else entirely.

There were no worshippers or rows of blue chairs. There was no stage or band, none of the wood panelling around the edge of the room. There were none of the things that Terry had pointed her camera at as she captured a feel of this place for her brother, Butch. All that could be seen was a swathe of buttery gold, with a thick ridge running through the centre, like the vein of a feather, close up.

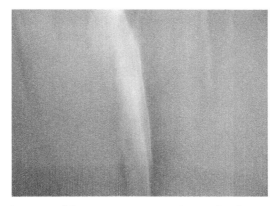

The next shot was like a progression from the first. It had the same buttery gold background, only now what looked like tongues of golden flame danced their way across it.

She leaned over and toggled the shots. 'See, the wings are closed here... and here, they're open.'

It was as if the vein was bunched-up stage curtains that opened in the second picture to reveal the flames.

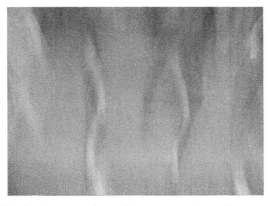

Puzzled, I looked around me for some point of connection between the pictures and our surroundings. But nothing looked even remotely similar to what I was looking at.

By the fourth shot in the sequence, the tongues of flame had become translucent, with the auditorium wall visible through them. By the fifth, fuzzy backs of heads could be seen. There was a man with a child in his arms, shot with purple streaks. I could see the stage below, with guitars and drums, and the screen with song lyrics, behind the band. After that, everything looked normal, as if the weird pictures had never been.

Going through the pictures again brought no answers. Of course they could be the result of a glitch in Terry's camera. Yet, inside my head, a little voice was reminding me that everything about tonight had been unexpected and unprecedented. And, okay, yes, supernatural.

Was it beyond belief that the waves of love that had felt so real I wanted to reach out and grasp them could have been captured and manifested in these pictures?

'Maybe so,' I said eventually, handing it back to her. 'Can we go up to the Prayer Tower now?'

'Sure.'

We headed for the door.

Unlike me, Terry hadn't forgotten the man who shook hands with us at the start of the service. She asked about him at the Information Desk in the foyer. The woman there shook her head. Terry turned to a cluster of people, chatting nearby. Her description of him drew blank faces there, too.

I was surprised; he'd acted like this was his place.

'I think Jesus himself came to greet us,' Terry said, as we stepped out of the basement church into the chilly shopping mall.

It was a nice notion but a bit far-fetched, I thought.

2.

We waited under stark, white neon to ride up to the Prayer Tower. I was still tingling all over but also feeling washed out, as if I'd had a good cry.

Eventually, steel doors shuddered open. A smell of engine oil and stale clothing wafted out. They opened again at the top floor of the building to reveal Jerusalem twinkling through a picture window, like fairyland at our feet.

We joined a dozen or so people, sitting in a large, loose circle under dimmed lights. I did not know what we were waiting for or what to expect. I had never been to a Prayer Tower before.

'Hi, I'm Chanelle.'

A young woman in jogging pants sank down at our feet in a limber position that spoke of ballet. There was a still quality about her that I immediately found engaging.

I slithered off my chair to join her on the floor.

Terry did the same. 'The Holy Spirit came upon my friend tonight. This is her first Christian experience.'

I was not very happy with her words. She spoke as though I'd already bought something when I felt I was still only window-shopping. I needed some time to think things through.

Foremost in my mind was how a defection to Christianity could turn me into a leper in my Jewish life. My family would view me as a traitor, the members of the South East London Women's New Moon Group that I myself set up would throw up their hands in horror and I was pretty sure my congregation would expel me.

A Star of David hung from Chanelle's neck. I wondered if she was Jewish. Probably not, I decided. Terry always wore one and she wasn't.

'What's your name?' Her accent was South African.

'Bobbie.'

She looked at me levelly and I found myself telling her, 'My marriage fell apart after my husband couldn't cope with me getting sick. My kids are all grown up. I've been hoping, through this trip to Israel, to find a purpose for my life.'

'You will dance again,' she said. Laying a hand on my shoulder, she began to pray for me.

Terry laid a hand on my other shoulder.

Chanelle asked God to allow me to trust and wait for His sign to show me my path. She finished, 'Please, Lord, take this woman as your obedient bride and give her rest. And, when the time is right for her, bless her with a new, earthly husband.'

Where had this come from? A new husband, or even a boyfriend, was not on my agenda right now. Since the break-up of my marriage, I'd found it impossible to go out with a man.

In the last month, I'd worked up to arranging two coffee dates through an internet dating site. Both were disasters. Unsmiling and ill at ease, I had grilled the men like I was interviewing them for a job. I had no idea how to behave on a date.

After the second fiasco, I cancelled my membership. A pop-up protested that it still had two months to run: was I sure? Yes, yes, yes.

Oblivious to my amazement, Chanelle swivelled her legs around and sat cross-legged. After considering me for a moment, she opened the bible on her lap. It was weighty and well-worn, with blocks of yellow highlighter and ballpoint pen scribbles across the pages.

Her hair hung down in long curtains as she read Psalm 37, a psalm of King David. It was quite long but she made no apology for that. I enjoyed what it said.

'*Trust in the Lord and do good, dwell in the land and enjoy safe pasture.*'

Also: '*Delight yourself in the Lord and he will give you the desires of your heart.'*

I wondered what the desires of my heart really were. Though I put on a brave face of managing alone, I had to admit that, deep down, I wanted to feel valued by someone dear to me. Throughout my marriage, and particularly through my darkest years, my ex had managed to make me feel the opposite. I yearned to be treasured, like the woman of Proverbs 31: *Her children arise and call her blessed, her husband also and he praises her.*

Chanelle read, '*Commit your way to the Lord, trust in Him and he will do this.'*

There was that word 'trust' again, a hard thing to do.

And 'commit'. I had trembled tonight during the worship, my heart had been moved, I had felt compelled. Even so, inside the barriers were still up. The idea of switching camps on the strength of a fuzzy feeling defied logic. I was not the sort of woman to throw herself headlong into something.

'*Be still before the Lord and wait patiently for him.'*

It would be good to be like Chanelle, calm and unhurried, to speak in a voice that was soft and even, to radiate kindness.

She closed her eyes. Her lips moved. She thumbed through her bible to the New Testament Book of Luke.

'I want to read you the Virgin Mary's song of celebration,' she said. 'She was thanking God for what the Holy Spirit had sent her — the baby Jesus in her womb. Mary was a brave woman. She wasn't married and would have faced disapproval on every side. She could even have been stoned.'

This was a second reference to babies in less than an hour. Perhaps Chanelle chose this text because of the baby shoot of faith inside me. Or perhaps she was aware of the disapproval I would have to deal with, if I became a Christian.

As she read, I imagined Mary, praying on her knees, as Christians do, (though, come to think of it, she would have been Jewish), filled with both joy and fear, as I was now.

'*For the Mighty One has done great things for me.'*

Was He doing great things for me, too? The idea that I might be that special to Him was new and exciting.

Chanelle closed her bible and prayed quietly for a moment. 'I think what you need is to be wrapped in a cloak.'

A surge of joy and wonder went through me. 'A cloak is very meaningful to me! Cloaks come up twice in the biblical Book of Ruth. She's very dear to my heart. Ruth is my Hebrew name. I love her loyalty and perseverance.'

More than this, I'd spent a large part of my time here in Israel gathering material for my final major project of a Certificate in Graphic Design I was taking at London's University of the Arts: I was going to layout and illustrate the Book of Ruth.

I'd photographed the landscapes Ruth might have walked through on her journey from Moab and checked out her lifestyle of 1000 years Before the Common Era at the Israel Museum.

Chanelle nodded and smiled, seemingly not the least bit surprised to have come up with a suggestion that was so meaningful to me. She got to her feet, hitched up her tracksuit bottoms and went off to look for the cloak she had in mind.

As I waited, I thought about cloaks in the Book of Ruth. When she first met Boaz, who would become her redeemer and husband, he asked God to spread His protective cloak — sometimes translated as 'wings' — over her. Later, when things between them seemed to be stalling, she went to him at the threshing floor and asked him to spread his cloak over her. By this, she meant she wanted him to marry her.

Cloaks still cover Jewish brides today. When my eldest son, Jeremy, married, he planed wooden poles and draped his prayer shawl over them. During the ceremony, he and his Canadian bride, Alicia, stood together underneath it. The prayer shawl symbolised that he was taking her under his protective wings.

It struck me that the two cloak prayers in Ruth, one for God's protection and one for marriage, were echoed in the twofold prayer Chanelle had prayed over me tonight.

She returned after a short search with a beautiful satin cloak the colour of the vivid green mineralised waters of the Dead Sea.

Across the Dead Sea, a few days previously, I had gazed at the mauve mountains of Moab, Ruth's homeland, in present-day Jordan. I had imagined her and Naomi, her mother-in-law, picking their way down one of the steep pack trails that hugged the gullies. Beside them, thundering waters, swollen from the winter rains, rushed down to the lowest place on earth.

Crossing over to where I stood, whether via the Jordan River shallows or by means of the ferry that once conveyed travellers across the Dead Sea, would mark the first stage in their journey to a new life and new hope.

Chanelle draped the cloak over me, shutting out the light. 'There.'

I might have been at the bottom of the sea myself, for all the muffled sounds about me.

She patted my shoulder. 'You just stay there, nice and cosy.'

As I sat in the dark, initially feeling a little foolish and wondering how long I was supposed to do this for, a creeping sensation began to inch through my body. All the scars from all the surgery I had began to ache. It was the strangest thing, as if every dead or damaged part of me was coming to life again. It was a good ache. It made me want to cry.

Chapter 2

1.

It was autumn, 1997. I was forty-five years old. I had just returned from a fitness class. No one else was home that afternoon. My husband — we'll call him Seth — was at the office. My eldest, Jeremy, 23, was away, working in Switzerland. Simon, 18, was away at school. Tania, 12, was at school locally. I took a shower.

As I let the hot water massage away the tension, I stopped, freeze-frame. There was a lump in my right breast, just below the nipple.

I washed the soap off my legs and feet and went back to it. Still there.

It was still there, too, when I put my bra on: a lump about the size of a plum. The lump of panic in my throat was the same size.

'We'll just take a peak,' the consultant said and slotted me in for day surgery.

His hand-out said I might feel groggy afterwards. I shouldn't drive or take any major decisions for twenty-four hours. But I lay in the hospital bed afterwards, feeling fine, a little light-headed, maybe.

My consultant came in. 'Mind if I sit on the bed?'

I hoisted myself onto my elbows and nodded, pleased. I'd had him down as stuffy and here he was being chummy.

'We have the results of the frozen section,' he said.

'Oh, yes?' I hadn't expected to know today.

'I'm afraid the lump is cancerous.'

Seth and I exchanged looks.

'The normal treatment is mastectomy,' he continued.

I found my voice. 'That's ludicrous!'

Later, as I waited for Seth to bring the car round to the front entrance of the clinic, I watched rooks flocking to a great, wizened oak, its leaves streaked with orange. High above me in the blue sky was a plane the size of a fly, with a long, white tail.

How come the world hadn't stopped?

2.

My treatment began with chemotherapy. Every dose landed me in hospital.

'It must be working well,' the nurses said cheerfully.

Starting with chemo was a bid to keep my breast, I also cut out salt and generally improved my diet. I went in for all sorts of therapies — aromatherapy, reflexology, even hypnotherapy. I had counselling, I meditated. Every day, I visualised my white cells as seagulls, pecking away at a putrid pile of fish on a beach, my cancer.

Two weeks after my first treatment, I had a fever. My pain threshold plummeted. Even a page of a book falling onto a scab on my thumb made me groan.

I lay on my bed and visualised my beach. The sun was beating down on my putrid fish but where were my seagulls? There were just a few of them, gliding overhead, with no strength to land.

The hospital told me to come in. My white cell count was down and I was admitted. I told myself they gave me an isolation room with triple glazing, a hatch to pass my food through and ferocious air conditioning because they were short of beds.

I moped in the chair, reluctant to see myself as the patient and own the bed. I decided to visit the chapel but found the red and blue rugs of the Islamic area cosier than its white walls and hard benches.

A nurse berated me when I returned. 'Did no one tell you your white cell count is low?'

'Yeah, it's a bit down.'

'Your neutrophils are all the way down to 18%.'

That sounded bad.

She stuck a needle in my backside and the door sucked closed behind her. I pulled up the covers and sighed, my spirits in free fall.

Closing my eyes, I returned to my seashore. The sun glowed thinly as I sent my sickly gulls up to the cliff to nest. Self-healing would have to go on hold, pending re-enforcements.

Out of nowhere, a huge, golden crab came side-stepping. It latched onto my putrid fish and began stuffing itself with great pincers. Tears of relief welled up and roll down my cheeks as I watched it do the work I couldn't.

I was sure God had sent me this crab. Thank You.

A week later, my white cell count was robust and my tumour had shrunk by half.

Half way through the chemotherapy, Terry came to visit me. I had been looking forward to seeing her and was most frustrated when she arrived to find me stuck in hospital. Although there were planned hospitalisations throughout this period, this one was unexpected. I needed a blood transfusion. This time it was my red cell count that was way down.

I recovered and we had a good visit, with walks in the countryside and even a day trip to France. We had established a pattern of regular visits, as well as holidays together, over the years that drew us ever closer as friends.

By the end of the course of chemo, the lump was gone.

I thought my consultant might look a bit more cheerful. 'We'll do a scan and another biopsy and see what they throw up.'

I'd had enough throwing up.

'Champagne?' Seth suggested that evening.

'Better wait for the results.'

'You'll be fine.'

He always said that.

After stray cancer cells, known as foci, were found, my consultant recommended a wider excision. When that wasn't enough, he recommended a mastectomy.

Now I was angry.

Seth tried to smooth things over. 'We'll go abroad afterwards ? get some sun together.'

'In a bikini?'

'You'll be back to normal in no time.'

'I'll never be normal again.'

I realised that I had no choice but to let my surgeon take his pound of flesh.

I surged back from the anaesthesia with my teeth chattering. A silver blanket was wrapped about me to try and get my temperature back up. I had gone into shock.

Women I met who were already on the road to recovery thought it no big deal to lose a breast.

It was a big deal to me.

Seth thought of me as a Poor Thing. He would never again grope me as I stood at the kitchen sink.

My histology found no foci this time.

'And none in the lymph nodes, either,' my consultant said.

'You mean I'll survive?'

'You have an excellent outlook.' He picked up his pen. 'We'll just mop up any stray cells with a course of radiotherapy.'

'But you just said...'

'Can't be too careful.'

Yet again, my heart sank. Cancer seemed to have me and wouldn't let me go.

They gave me a pink jellyfish to slip into my bra. It had a life of its own, outside of my control. It would go missing and turn up in strange places. One day, as I walked around my mare, grooming her and picking out her feet, I realised it had thrown itself into the steaming pile of khaki-coloured poo behind her back legs.

There was no question whether or not I would be having reconstruction, merely how soon. They told me I would have to wait while the wound caused by radiotherapy healed.

During those months, Seth's sister began radiotherapy for breast cancer. The plan was that she would keep her breast. In France, where she lived, they claimed good results from radiotherapy as an alternative to mastectomy.

'It will be hard for her, as a single woman,' Seth commented, out of the blue, one day. 'Her skin will be stained from radiotherapy.'

I had developed a brown, rectangular stain the size of a small paperback book, following my own treatment. But it was on skin that was taut across my ribcage, like a boy's. Hers might be less visible.

'Of course,' he mused, 'it would have been worse if she'd needed a mastectomy.'

I frowned. His meaning was unclear. Was it that my sister-in-law would have felt bad about herself, following a mastectomy, or that no man would want her?

'No man would want her with one breast!' His tone implied that this was glaringly obvious.

I was deeply wounded. He couldn't have stated more plainly that he considered me hideous.

And why not? I thought I was hideous, too.

He had told me the story of his first lover, who had only one arm. He'd been repulsed by her sleeping with her, I asked, 'If I'd had to go through all this in our early days, would you have left me?'

I was playing the devil's advocate. It backfired on me.

'Maybe.'

3.

As I watched a video on reconstruction put out by the charity Breast Cancer Care, I recognised a glamorous volunteer on the catwalk of their mastectomy fashion show: I had just read the report of her death in their magazine. She was about my age.

I felt vulnerable and was comforted when Seth slumped into the armchair beside me to watch along with me. It was great that he wanted to learn about mastectomy and the reconstruction methods I was reviewing. Reconstruction was now my urgent and total preoccupation.

However, when the video finished, he began flipping channels and landed on a station showing soft porn.

'Ah, good,' he said. 'Let's look and see if she's normal.'

He couldn't understand why I fell apart.

Though I'd never be normal again, I could opt for the Rolls Royce of available reconstructive methods. My plastic surgeon could use my belly flesh to build me an authentic-looking, new breast. The problem was this method was a lot riskier than other methods.

I shared my concerns with a dear friend. 'The surgery is so major but the results, at best, will be a compromise.'

'Not a compromise,' Valerie countered, 'but the best, the very best you can do from your current perspective of one-breasted woman. It's only a compromise if you look at it from the position of who you were before. You need to say goodbye to that person in order to start afresh.'

I never really considered the surgery might fail. Somewhere in the back of mind, I had the idea God owed me, after I'd worked so hard to save my breast and failed at that.

My plastic surgeon said he wanted to make sure the artery he would use hadn't been compromised by the radiotherapy.

After the arteriogram, I was told not to move, except to go to the toilet, until the following day.

Seth picked me up. We drove home in silence. He seemed gloomy, as if he'd had enough of my being ill and this was too much. He was plain grumpy over supper.

He made up the sofa bed for me downstairs and went up to bed at nine. It was the first day of Channel Four's Breast Cancer Week. I watched a programme about two women who were cycling across the USA, fundraising for breast cancer and meeting local sufferers, along the way.

The programme ended with a surprise whammy. It revisited where everybody was today. Though some were well, others had died. Some whose lymph nodes had been clear like mine had developed secondaries and were now very sick.

I called up to Seth to come down and comfort me.

'I'm in bed,' he said. He refused to budge, no matter how much I pleaded and cried.

I wept in my lonely bed that night.

This, and other events, such as yelling at me when I was returned late to my hospital room after surgery, chipped away at us. But it was how he was when I was at my lowest ebb, when my reconstructive surgery went badly wrong, that would change my whole perspective on who we were as a couple.

4.

Three weeks before my surgery, I made the mad move of buying a new horse. Dizzy was a bright bay thoroughbred gelding with a reversed question-mark, like a dribble of white paint, down his nose.

I loved him.

Figuratively-speaking, I took him into hospital with me. He was a vision of the well and active person I was about to become again.

My side room on the eighth floor at St. Thomas's Hospital looked out at Big Ben and tourists on Westminster Bridge or in boats on the Thames. A lone seagull hovered outside my window. I didn't like it. It reminded me too much of a lone seagull I had seen just before I was admitted to hospital with a dangerously low white cell count.

Placing my silicone prosthesis in its box, I took a long last look at my flat chest and winking scar in the mirror — there were eyelashes where the stitches had been. Why was I doing this? The answer seemed to be because I had to.

Calm was on me as I was wheeled down early the next morning to the operating theatre. It was Thursday. The next I knew it was Friday morning and I was in the Recovery Room. Seth wasn't there. He wasn't even in the hospital.

My new mound looked beautiful. Even though it was mauve and congested, it was a lovely, natural shape. I lay back, content, and let the procession of staff do what they had to.

My plastic surgeon came in, looked at my new breast and sucked in his breath. 'It was a long operation,' he said. 'Nine hours. We'll see how things go.'

A haematoma, a very big clot, formed. I had further surgery the next morning to ease it. As soon as I woke up, I snuck a peak. It was still a great shape, though blotchy and dark.

My lungs hurt. A physiotherapist came and taught me how to take a breath in short stages. I kept dozing off, only to be woken by the alarm on the oxygen monitor. My breathing was too shallow.

I have been given heparin to stop further blood clots. My drains were filling up fast. A drain in the corner got overlooked. Suddenly, it was overflowing with blood. My sheets were bloody, too. Nurses talked over me as they shifted me around to change them. They kept coming in and out, checking things and shaking their heads.

They rigged me up for a blood transfusion.

'Your haemoglobin count is under six,' said the young Nigerian doctor who stayed at my bedside all night.

Coldly, I considered the possible outcome of all this. It would be a smooth and painless death. I would just get weaker until I fell asleep. That wasn't scary at all, really. Meanwhile, there were things I could do. I could use the tips the physio gave me to stay calm and breathe. I could focus on my pulse, nice and slow and regular.

The doctor brought a hypodermic and very slowly administered an antidote to the Heparin, as the Australian nurse who also stayed all night by me monitored my blood pressure. The atmosphere was tense as it went in but, job done, they smiled at one another, looking relieved.

At 3 a.m., they called my surgeon. My mound had become cool to the touch.

A nurse phoned Seth the next morning and told him I was going down for further surgery.

But he wasn't there when I came to with a howl at the end of this third operation in hardly as many days, this time to remove my beautiful replacement breast.

There were only the Recovery Room nurses, chatting across me about the price of second-hand cars. When I asked them to call up to the ward for my husband, I learned he was not even in the building.

He had stayed home.

He shrugged when I asked him why. 'The nurse said come after. I didn't realise.'

He didn't stay long. That night was the World Cup Soccer Final. He wasn't about to miss watching that.

Broken-hearted, I concluded it made no odds to him whether I lived or died.

The Breast Care Nurse came to offer sympathy for my lost mound. 'You'll need a focus for your anger, I'm sure,' she said.

'I think I'll blame God,' I replied.

'He's got broad shoulders,' she said. 'He can take it.'

A week later, I came home from hospital as empty as the mother leaving maternity with no baby.

Looking at the raw crater that remained, I thought myself repulsive. There was a similar gaping wound in my marriage.

5.

Six months later, my plastic surgeon rebuilt my breast by tunnelling muscle around from my back. It was a lot smaller than the other one. I returned to have an implant inserted, then again, so that a thick nodule of flesh between my 'breasts' could be excised.

The end result looked okay, like I'd been involved in a bad accident, maybe.

Things were getting back to normal when Dizzy suddenly decided to do a rodeo one day. I landed on my knees and broke my hip, which put me in a wheelchair for a while and on crutches a good deal longer.

I slipped on some wet floor tiles and the screws holding my broken bone in place were dislodged. After six months of wondering daily whether they would pierce the skin, my doctor judged it safe to remove them. The bone held and I escaped a hip replacement.

All told, I had thirteen rounds of surgery in three years.

6.

The next challenge in my series of woes was pulmonary embolisms, clots on the lung. I found myself bed-bound in an Irish hospital, having been taken ill while staying at a writers' retreat on the Beara Peninsular. I had to keep still and was only allowed to move to go to the bathroom. The danger was that a clot would dislodge and go to my heart, killing me.

The old ladies on the ward had names like Elizabeth, Hannah and Julia. Julia, in her nineties, smoked in the ladies' washroom but told the physiotherapist she'd given up. An old lady came and sat on the end of my bed and asked me where the pub was.

A younger woman had a cough and a breathing problem. After diapers on and lights out at eleven, her cough did the round of the ward and came back to her, over and over, throughout the night. I kept my hands over my ears and sang every Beatles song I could remember.

Between the building works in the room next door and the loud, nocturnal televisions of the patients, peace was absent.

Seth came towards the end of my first week there. The painful gasses test the doctor carried out on my artery made tears roll down. I asked Seth to get me a piece of chocolate. To my amazement, he refused and told me, 'You're behaving like a spoilt child.'

Supper had been poor and served at four but that was not the point. The point was I craved something sweet in my life.

Tests showed up multiple pulmonary embolisms. Seth would not believe me when I told him the risks so the kind and friendly nurse, who accompanied me to Cork and back in the ambulance, explained them to him.

Eventually, I began to sleep better, sitting leaning back against five, heaped pillows, oblivious to the vacuum cleaner, the calling of the nurses to one another, the Mexican-wave coughing...

The journey home was awful. I was repatriated with oxygen and a nurse.

Though the Warfarin— a rat poison — I was prescribed took it out of me, gradually I was able to go for walks, though hills were still a problem. I couldn't keep up with my father-in-law, who was in his eighties.

I always wanted to know where I was going and how long I'd be, in order to store up sufficient reserves of energy ahead of time.

The family travelled to Paris at Christmastime, 2001. On Christmas Day, when we went out for lunch, I found myself sitting outside alone in the searing cold and rain, as the cigarette smoke which filled the restaurant was choking me.

Neither Seth, nor anyone else, came out to see how I was. I was two months on from my lung clots diagnosis in October. Sitting on the sidewalk on a hard-backed chair the waiter brought out for me, I got a very strange look from some people leaving their apartment building.

When my fiftieth birthday came, my kids wanted to take me out for a surprise. This idea filled me with dread. I was massively relieved when we went to a fancy restaurant in my area and not up to Central London, where I might be overtaken by exhaustion.

After this, things were pretty bad between Seth and me.

Finally I got shingles, which was agony.

I didn't deserve any of it. I raged at God's injustice.

Chapter 3

1.

After the Prayer Tower, we walked back to our guesthouse just outside the Jaffa Gate. All the way, Terry speculated about the meaning of what she was now confidently calling the angels in her camera.

The pictures were intriguing.

It struck me that the colour and texture of my beautiful *tallit* prayer shawl and its matching *kippah*, or skull cap, was the exact same buttery gold silk as these pictures.

It was made especially for my adult *Bat Mitzvah*, in 2003. I marked my return to health by confirming my status as a 'Daughter of the Commandment' on my 51st birthday.

I wanted my prayer shawl to be feminine, bright and cheerful. So I rejected the customary blue stripe on white fabric styles echoed in the Israeli flag, in favour of commissioning a U.S. fibre artist to create the *tallit* cloak she named *Chag Aviv*, or 'Spring Festival'.

Flowers and gambolling lambs were painted above a mosaic fabric collage of reds, greens and browns, representing the fertile earth, across the bottom. Two of my *tallit*'s four tasselled corners were embroidered with spring flowers, a third with a dove of peace and the fourth with a fish. I wondered about this, knowing it to be a Christian symbol, but my designer said it represented God's eye that never closes.

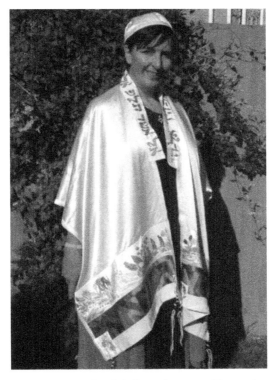

Picture: *Jewish Renaissance Magazine*

Friends and relatives, Jewish and non-Jewish, looked back at me as I stood on the synagogue dais, wearing my prayer shawl and skull cap. Some were members of my *Rosh Chodesh*, New Moon, Women's Group. In the front row sat Jeremy and Alicia, who was heavily pregnant, — I was about to become a grandmother for the first time — my second son, Simon, now 23, and my daughter, Tania, 19. They would read liturgy and poetry I had picked, to make the service personal and meaningful.

I'd asked Seth to say a few words on my special day to celebrate my survival. In my dreams, he would stand up and tell the congregation that I meant something to him.

'No,' came his blunt answer.

Bewildered, I asked, 'Why?'

'It's not my thing,' was all the explanation I received.

My Bat Mitzvah formed part of the regular, Saturday morning service. I read the *Torah* portion designated for that week from a weighty scroll, inscribed with the first five books of the bible in

Hebrew. There were no vowels, only consonants. My Hebrew was very weak. I had spent a lot of time with my coach preparing for this.

First, I gave my *drasha*, or speech, about the passage which dealt with the cleansing of a house from 'leprosy'.

Initially, I had found this portion from tinder-dry Leviticus uninspiring. As I went deeper into it, however, I began to draw parallels between what my body had been through and the treatment prescribed for a sick house: if thorough cleaning and keeping an eye on it did not work, the infected section was to be cut out and carried away to an unclean place, outside of the city.

We might pooh-pooh such rituals as superstition, I argued, but was what we called science really very different?

It was an effective speech but not a Godly one. I gave God none of the credit for healing me.

He was not really invited to my *Bat Mitzvah* at all.

Chapter 4

1.

Even though so much had been churned up inside my head by my experience at the church and in the Prayer Tower that evening, I slept soundly.

I awoke the next morning to find Terry, dressed and ready to go, sitting at the foot of my bed. Her camera was in her hand.

'I've been awake all night,' she said, 'walking around the reception area. I have to find a rabbi to look at these pictures.'

'But we're leaving for Tel Aviv today,' I said. Today would be our last day together. Tomorrow, she was flying back to Canada. The day after that, I was returning to England.

'I want to show my pictures to a rabbi from King of Kings,' she said, with a determined look that I knew well.

King of Kings, or *Melech HaMelechim*, was the name of the church we had attended the previous evening.

I wondered why she kept saying 'rabbi' instead of 'pastor', but I didn't have the jive for the world of Jewish Christian believers and I was not about to challenge her on her vocabulary.

I tried another tack. 'Do you think we'll even find anybody there on a Monday morning?'

She sent me an owlish look.

'Okay,' I capitulated, throwing back the covers and getting to my feet. 'After breakfast, we'll go to the Old City and get that book I wanted, then we'll head back to King of Kings and ask at the office there... if it's open.'

The book in question was *Il Rotollo di Ruth*, (The Scroll of Ruth). A bible bookstore just inside the Jaffa Gate had it, in Italian only. Intended for Catholic priests visiting from the Vatican, the bookseller explained, it offered a line by line translation of the Book of Ruth from the original Hebrew. I had hesitated about buying it because I had almost no Italian. But I knew French and that was similar. I decided I wanted it, regardless.

'Good,' Terry said. 'That's a plan.'

As we later came out of the bookstore with *Il Rotollo di Ruth* in my hand, a white Mercedes taxi drew up, alongside of us. The driver hailed Terry. 'Hello, Sister!'

I recognised him.

'*Shalom*, brother!' she cried, waving her arms wildly in greeting.

We had met him the previous Friday. Curiously, Ruth was present on that occasion also.

I knew straight away that the life-size, painted wooden statue in the antique shop window was her by the bundle of sheaves she carried under her arm. The shop was shut for the Sabbath, so I took my photos from outside, through the plate glass window. I could see the reflection of a white Mercedes taxi as it came to a halt in the road behind us.

The driver wound down the passenger window and hailed us in typical Jerusalem style. 'Where you want to go? I know a nice shop of friends. Great souvenirs. Beautiful jewellery. I take you there.'

'No, thank you,' I told him and turned back to Ruth. She was dressed in shades of ruddy brown. She looked happy.

But Terry, who was always everybody's friend, leaned on the car window and said, 'We're looking for a community that used to worship at the YMCA.'

We had just come from the surprisingly ornate, colonial building of the Jerusalem YMCA. I had gazed at grandiose arches and pillars as Terry asked the man at reception about King of Kings — she had attended one of their services on a previous visit and enjoyed it — but they had moved on, she learned. The helpful receptionist phoned everybody he could think of but no one seemed to have any idea where they now met.

She came away disappointed.

'You mean *Melech haMelechim*?' the taxi driver asked.

'Yes!' Terry threw up her arms in delight.

'You wanna go there?'

'No,' I said.

'Yes,' she said.

'You are a believer?' His face lit up. 'King of Kings is my congregation!'

'It is?'

'Sister!' He got out of his car and came around to hug her. He was about forty-five, with dark hair, eyes and skin, and a ready smile.

'Brother!' Terry hugged him back.

Oh-oh. I fiddled with my camera, hoping he would not be coming to me next. I did not want a hug from some rip-off-merchant cabbie. I did not want to be whisked away to shop for souvenirs at his 'friends'. And I thought Terry naive for being so unguarded around him.

But, after introducing himself as Adam and telling us where and when King of Kings held their meetings in English, he got back in his cab. With a cheery wave and a, 'God bless you, sisters!', he drove away.

My pictures of the statue of Ruth turned out almost as odd as Terry's angel pictures. Superimposed over the Reaper Maid of 1000 years BCE, as she stood amongst the antique clocks and mahogany desks, was the reflection of Adam's shiny, white Mercedes.

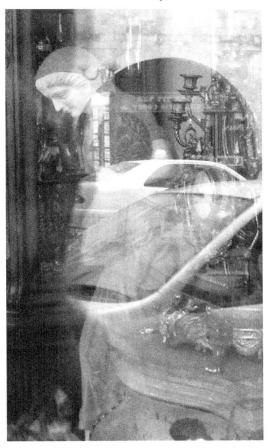

Now here he was again, like the genie in the lamp, outside a Jaffa Gate bible bookshop.

Terry leaned through the passenger window and told him, 'We're looking for a rabbi from King of Kings congregation.'

'I can help you with that, Sister!'

'You can?'

Of course he could. He could help us find an elephant, if we wanted one.

I stood a little way off, with my arms folded in front of me, convinced that this little search would cost us a heap of money.

'I know a nice shop of friends. You go there and drink coffee,' he said, pointing to a dark, little store in the corner of the cobbled square. 'I arrange what you want. I find the rabbi.'

As Adam drove away, Terry headed across to the store. I trailed after her, wishing we were on our way to Tel Aviv, as we had said we would be.

We crossed the threshold and the manager launched into action, brusquely sending out for coffee. He then showed us carpets and souvenirs. They were beautiful and expensive. Had I wandered in here of my own volition, I might have enjoyed looking at them.

*****

Dolls' house sized cups of Turkish coffee appeared on a great, bronze platter. Terry had gone outside when Adam returned, so I found myself sitting alone in a low chair, sipping the sweet, muddy liquid. To watch them through the shop window was like watching t.v. He was talking on his cell phone. She was fidgeting as she stood before him, hardly able to contain all that dynamic energy I usually found so attractive in her. Yet what they were doing involved me: they were going to whisk me away somewhere I didn't know.

With bad grace, I bought a silver bracelet for my daughter. It had a Turkish, filigree look to it. Only later did I concede that it was actually quite pretty and not expensive.

I escaped from the manager and came outside to find Terry showing Adam the angel pictures on her digital display.

'Halleluyah, sister!' he cried. 'Praise the Lord!'

He sounded so phony.

'Come on, Bobbie,' Terry said. 'He's going to take us to a rabbi so I can show him the photos. And he'll drive us to Tel Aviv afterwards.'

'Which rabbi? Where are we going?'

'Someone he knows. Adam is part of the messianic community here. You know, Jews who believe in Jesus.'

Even though Terry had been to Israel a number of times before, she clearly did not understand the Middle Eastern Jewish ways like I did. My experience was more than that of a returning tourist. My former husband was an Egyptian Jew. Throughout my marriage, I had dealings with North African business owners. Though their talk would often be can-do and special-for-you, the end price would not seem special for me at all. Allowing ourselves to be carried off on a hunt for a nebulous 'rabbi' was just asking to be exploited.

She tilted her head quizzically. 'What's the matter?'

'We don't know this person,' I hissed.

She looked as if she felt sorry for me. 'You think everybody's out to trick us.'

She took a deep breath and led me away from the cab. 'Bobbie, please wait for me at the guesthouse. I'm going with him.'

'No,' I protested. 'I couldn't do that.'

'It's okay,' she said gently. 'I'll be fine. Have a cup of coffee and have the bags ready to go as soon as I return.'

'But I...'

'Wait for me. Have a cup of coffee.'

'Alright, then.' I conceded. 'So, I'll see you later?'

'Yes.' She smiled.

'Right.' I gave a half wave as I walked away, feeling both excluded and indignantly self-righteous.

Ten minutes later, I was back at the guesthouse. I stood beneath the Israeli flag that furled above our balcony and looked back at the walls of the Old City and the Jaffa Gate, where we just were, wondering what Terry was doing now.

Throughout this trip, she had shown me only patience and tolerance as I pursued whatever interested me. She deserved better from me than to let her go off on her own with strangers.

It was time to check out. I returned my key and sat in reception, surrounded by cases and bags, as if guarding them were my task, as if by doing this, I could somehow compensate for abandoning my friend.

The guesthouse was hosting some kind of armed forces conference. The delegates must have broken for lunch because hoards of camel-coloured uniforms were spilling out of the café and filling the foyer. I was surrounded by young Israeli conscripts with complexions as dark as dates, all talking in Hebrew.

I willed them to part and reveal a frenzy of blond hair, coming in my direction.

I occupied myself with idling through the sequence of shots on my own camera's digital display. I had taken countless pictures of biblical-looking scenes, like the view of vineyards and cedars from Oasis of Peace, where we had stayed, in the foothills of Jerusalem. This village, school, conference centre and guesthouse, run jointly by Jews and

Arabs, was founded by a Christian Dominican brother, whose dream was to create a place where 'My people will live in peaceful dwelling places, in secure homes, in undisturbed places of rest.' (Isaiah 32:18).

Many of my pictures were from a coach excursion to the Galilee that Terry had signed us up for. With her, I had visited Christian sites like Nazareth or Capernaum that, as a Jew, I had never seen before. At Capernaum, Terry was excited to learn that archaeologists had discovered the remains of a first century synagogue beneath the fourth century one already being excavated. Potentially, this was the very one where Jesus would have worshipped.

How strange to think of Jesus attending synagogue. It had never really registered with me before that he was Jewish.

Three hours dragged by. I was squirming with guilt and worry. Finally, Terry appeared. She was white and glowing like Moses, coming down from the mountain. She picked up a bag to carry outside. Though she moved purposefully, she did not speak. She seemed to be in some inner world that kept a secret smile hovering on her lips.

Adam was nowhere to be seen but his cab was outside. She hugged the tall stranger who brought her back as if they were old friends and he left, refusing to take a penny from her. A 'brother' of his appeared to drive us to Tel Aviv.

All the way there, a drive of an hour or more, she hardly said a word and her responses to my own conversation openers were monosyllabic. This was so out of character that I didn't know what to make of it all.

I bit my lip and did not mention the wait or reproach her for any of the terrible scenarios my imagination had inflicted on me.

2.

Why our Tel Aviv hotel was so hard to find, I do not know. Our driver drove around for ages, asking people for directions. After we finally checked in, I pulled back the bedroom curtains and discovered we were just across the road from the seafront.

By now, the sun was a great red ink blot, inches above the Mediterranean. We had spent the whole of our last day together in Jerusalem.

We went out to eat and found an American diner with Russian waitresses and a Hebrew-speaking clientele. Though it was March, it was warm enough here, on the coast, to sit outside on the terrace, under a jaunty parasol.

Terry's face was still glowing. She continued to look like she was smirking. I grew antsy. I had earned some sharing, I felt, after being so noble after my long wait. Eventually, I told her as much.

Her eyes widened in surprise. She considered for a moment. Perhaps she was praying. 'Okay.'

A long pause followed.

'Well?' I felt like kicking her in the shins.

Haltingly, she began to tell me that the rabbi she had met with had confirmed the pictures in her camera were of angels.

I was surprised to hear this. But, then, what did I know of angels?

'I'm nobody but God has sent me angels.' She gave her head a shake. 'Wow! He's taken me at my word and claimed me as His girl.'

She fell silent again after the waitress brought out pasta.

'Go on,' I said, eventually.

'The rabbi prophesied over me. I have an important mission for the faith.'

It didn't seem fair. I was the one who was free and available, whereas she had a husband to look after, not to mention an eight-year old son from a late pregnancy at age 42.

'What kind of a mission?'

'I don't know… But, guess what, Bobbie? I'll be seeing a lot of light!'

I sighed. These sound bites were not her style at all. She was being exasperatingly cryptic for someone who more usually spouted long, involved stories.

Her lips were working. 'There's a rug. We're both on it.'

My face muscles tugged every which way to form a flabbergasted face. I hadn't the faintest idea what she was talking about. 'What do you mean, "on it"?'

A grin spread across her face. She nodded, smiling inside.

'What kind of a rug?'

Long after I had given up any hope of receiving an answer, she said, 'I only saw it for a minute, after the rabbi prayed over me. I can't remember the detail. We were riding horses. There were rabbits and deer…'

'How are we on a rug, riding horses?' I asked. 'You mean we're depicted on it?'

'Yes.'

Terry was prone to making a good story out of flimsy evidence. I guess my mind's eye imagined a portrait that bore some kind of generic resemblance to the two of us.

'And?' Despite my scepticism, I was eager to know more.

'I don't know.' An expression flashed across her face as she sighed and I understood that she was not being secretive to frustrate me. She was filled with fear. I assumed she didn't know what was okay to pass on and what was not.

Then she seemed to come to a decision. She leaned forward and told me everything, without pausing.

'Adam drove me to some kind of a warehouse,' she said. 'We went through a room where rolled-up rugs were piled like dropped scrolls. The place had a funny smell that make me think of Ali Baba's cave — oil and spices. Musty. We sat on hard-backed chairs in a dingy backroom. Adam introduced the rabbi when he came in. I put out my hand to shake his but he looked in the other direction.'

I knew all about this. Many Jewish men won't shake hands with a woman since she might be ritually unclean, i.e. menstruating.

'He sat down,' she continued. 'He was a big man with a beard. His body overflowed the chair. He brushed the street off his clothing and said, "*Ken?*" (Well?)

'I handed my camera to the guy who brought me back to the guesthouse this afternoon. His name's Yonaton. He was going to interpret because the rabbi spoke only Hebrew. When Yonaton showed him the pictures, the rabbi's face changed. He began talking very fast.'

'Was he actually from King of Kings' Hebrew congregation?' I asked.

But my attempt to authenticate the rabbi's credentials drew no response from Terry, whose eyes wore a glassy expression. She was back in the warehouse.

'"It's an angel!" Yonaton translated, getting excited, too. The rabbi threw up his hands. "He says that the angel is *Binyamin*!" Yonaton continued.'

Terry frowned. '"*Binyamin*?" I said, not understanding.

'"The tribe whose territory includes Jerusalem," he replied.

I understood *Binyamin*. 'That's Hebrew for Benjamin,' I said.

I'd never heard of an angel called Benjamin before. All I knew of Benjamin was that it was one of the twelve tribes of Judah's sons in the Bible.

'That's right, Bobbie. That's what they told me. "Praise the Lord!" Yonaton cried. They all got up and hugged one another. I got up and hugged Yonaton and Adam, too. I was blown away by it all. The rabbi sat down again, sweating and dabbing at his brow with a folded handkerchief, though it really wasn't hot in there — I still had my jacket on.'

I had finished my plate of pasta. As I pushed it away, Terry noticed that her own plate was untouched. She picked up her fork and took a few bites.

'Go on,' I said.

'The rabbi started speaking again and Yonaton translated. "He says that you should write down the names of your husband and children and the name of your friend who is travelling with you. We will pray for you at our meetings. We are five hundred people."

This last statement was reassuring. Whether or not this prophetic 'rabbi' was from King of Kings, he was at least in charge of a congregation.

'They brought me a pencil and a scrap of paper. My hand was shaking as I wrote the information down. "I don't understand what all this means," I told Yonaton. "Please ask the rabbi to tell me."

'The rabbi got to his feet again. He was swaying, with his eyes closed. His words came in short bursts as his big hands drew a wide circle. "Huge, it is huge," Yonaton translated. "But all in God's time. You must be patient. You will hear a little at a time, because it is huge."'

I cut in. 'What is huge?'

Terry blinked 'That's what I wanted to know. His answer was, "God will direct your feet through many doors. You will turn to the right and to the left. You will go through a bigger door and then a bigger door. The Lord will show you the way. It will be huge."

She closed her eyes. 'I closed my eyes. I could see myself going through doors. "Yes, yes," I said. "Thank you, Jesus. Whatever is required, I will do."'

Though I was still sceptical, I was enthralled by what I was hearing. The last part, about going through ever bigger doors, reminded me of a verse I knew from Isaiah: Whether you turn to the right or to the left, your ears will hear a voice behind you, saying, 'This is the way; walk in it.' (Isaiah 30:21)

'Yonaton was a really tall man, maybe six five,' she went on, 'But he dropped straight onto his knees and began to pray. He began shaking his head, as if he was seeing something wondrous. A smile spread across his face and he looked up to heaven. "Praise God," he said. "I see your home!"

'"My house in Canada?" I cried. "Yes! There are rabbits and deer all around it!" "That's exactly right!" I said. "Your home is... the target," he said. "The target?" I said. "Yes," he said, "the most important." "The centre?" I suggested.

'He was pleased when I said this. "Yes!" he cried. Then he frowned. "There are horses?" I told him that I had sold them.'

Anger flashed through Terry's eyes. She leaned towards me. 'Don was supposed to build stables for them but he never did. And he was supposed to ride with me. That didn't happen, either.'

I had never met Don, her husband of ten years, or their little boy, Lonnie. Neither had I seen her home in Eastern Canada. She moved back to her native New Brunswick from British Columbia, where she lived when we first met, around the same time that I was diagnosed with cancer.

During my treatment for that and the subsequent lung clots, I avoided long haul flights. My five-hour flight here to Israel was the longest plane journey I'd undertaken in years. However, Terry had visited me in England several times during that period.

She resumed her account. '"Now you have new horses!" Yonaton cried. He jumped to his feet and disappeared through the door we came in by. I stared after him. I had no idea what he meant or where he had gone.

'Adam, the cab driver, took over as interpreter. "Do not speak of any of this to untrustworthy people," he translated. "And do not use the power and authority given to you through this prophecy for personal gain."

'I told him "Okay."'

'Then Yonaton came back, carrying a rolled up rug. "Sister," he said, with a wide grin. (He has a mouthful of big, white teeth.) "You are going to be seeing a lot of light!" He unrolled the rug at my feet. I was amazed when I saw it.'

She leaned back in her chair.

Even in her trance-like, otherworldly state, I knew she was keeping me dangling.

'That's it?' I capitulated.

'That's it.'

'So what was it that was amazing?'

'It's really us. It's a hunting rug. We are both on it, hunting.'

'Is this a vision you had when you saw the rug?'

'Oh, no vision, Bobbie. The rug is real. It's really us.'

But for my bad attitude, I would have seen it for myself and made up my own mind about it. What a missed opportunity!

She frowned. 'Maybe you're fishing. I only saw it for a minute. You're doing this.' She made a harpooning gesture.

'Our likenesses are woven into it?'

'Yes. We're riding Arabian horses.'

'There are lots of rabbits and deer. There are other people on it, too, two men.'

I could not begin to imagine what such a rug might look like. 'Who are they?'

She shrugged. 'I don't know.'

It was quite dark now and a breeze was lifting. Lights had begun to twinkle up and down the promenade. I put on my cardigan and sighed. I liked black and white: none of this prophecy seemed to add up to anything concrete.

The rug was different. If we really were on it, not only was its existence miraculous, but also the fact that we had found it. Or it had found us.

I waved to the waitress to bring the bill.

Fumbling for her wallet, Terry threw in, almost as an aside, 'I think they're going to send it to me.'

3.

Angels, it seemed, were everywhere that evening. A stroll along the esplanade brought us to a massive, verdigris angel statue. After taking photos, we walked on to the cobbled streets of Old Jaffa. This quaint area is full of art galleries. They all seemed to have angel paintings on display.

We returned to our hotel around nine and sat in the lobby, a modest but comfortable space, with a wall-mounted TV that was mercifully set to silent. No one came in or out.

'It's like we're the only ones here,' Terry commented, with an air of mystery.

'No one else could have found it,' I replied.

We chatted with the receptionist, a man by the name of Bero. Terry's usual display of exuberant friendliness left me feeling like a cardboard cut-out. The man had naughty, dancing eyes that unnerved me. I thought he might be secretly laughing at us. Or he could be a letch.

I did not mean to be so mistrustful. It seemed I could only deal in stereotypes and viewed everyone as suspect.

He offered us mint tea. When he brought it, he pulled up a chair and joined us. He was about fifty years old, dark and small-framed.

'What time would you like breakfast in the morning?' he asked.

I looked at Terry. 'I'm easy,' I told her. 'You choose.'

'When would you like?' she asked.

'Seven?'

'Sure.'

Bero blinked approvingly. 'You are good friends?'

'Yes,' we answered in unison and smiled at one another.

'I see it. It is unusual for people to consider one another's wishes as you do. You are kind to one another.'

'We are,' Terry said.

'Yours is a very special friendship,' Bero said.

I nodded. Mutual respect, admiration and genuine liking had sustained us over the years.

I would have thought that everybody would love someone as fun as Terry was. Yet that had not been the case on a couple of occasions during this trip. When she took me to the Garden Tomb, a woman in the office had been sharp with her and looked down her nose, as if to say: *who are you to be so cheerful*? And at the Oasis of Peace Guesthouse, some men who struck up a conversation with us had stared at her peroxide hair and tight jeans, clearly missing the beautiful person inside.

'You are from different countries?'Bero said.

'I'm from New Brunswick in the Canadian Maritimes,' Terry volunteered.

She had shown me exactly where on a big, pioneer map of North America that happened to be pinned above our heads when we ate in a cowboy café in Arad, in the Negev Desert. The Province of New Brunswick lay on the Atlantic, sandwiched between Nova Scotia and Quebec and bordering the U.S. State of Maine. Firs and lakes were sketched in the wide spaces between the towns.

'Empty of people,' she had said, 'and, right now, deep in snow.'

Bero didn't ask me where I was from. Perhaps I looked too hostile. 'Do you like to ride horses?' he asked Terry, *à propos* of nothing.

Her eyes widened. She sent me a meaningful look. 'I do!'

He grinned. 'And do you like to hunt?'

Clearly, she thought he was in on whatever it was she was involved in. She elbowed me in the ribs, then flicked her wrist at him. 'Aw, you know!'

His questions were remarkably in line with the description she had just given me of the rug. However, that didn't necessarily mean he had any special knowledge. They were too broad and general to jump to that conclusion.

Bero smiled. His eyes twinkled. I was convinced he thought of himself as a player.

'Where are you from?' Terry asked him.

'Originally from Turkey.' He immediately deflected the conversation away from himself by asking me, 'You have had a good visit in Israel?'

'Yes.'

Covering my terseness, Terry described some of the places we had visited. 'It's been wonderful.'

'Are you happy to be returning home now?' He was looking at me.

I hadn't asked for a mint tea. I hadn't asked him to pull up a chair and ask me questions. Seeing my arms folded across my chest, Terry stepped in again. 'Yes, I am. I miss my husband and my little boy.'

'Ah.' His tone implied he knew all about them.

'And Bobbie is from London, England,' she said.

He turned to me. 'So what is your dream?'

I thought this was none of his business. If Terry hadn't been so obviously impressed by him, I would have said so. I shrugged noncommittally. 'Dunno.'

'I think I know what you really want.' It was his turn to sound mysterious.

'Really?'

Terry leaned forward. 'Do tell us.'

'Yes,' I said. 'Do tell me what I really really want.'

'What you both really want,' Bero said, '...is true love.' His blink was almost a wink.

'I'm married.' Terry seemed blithely unaware that her words could be interpreted as implying that marriage and true love were mutually exclusive.

I wondered how God could possibly give me a new husband as Chanelle had prayed? How could I love again, when all trust was gone?

Bero saw my cogs turning and, with a half nod, switched subject. 'You could fit in anywhere, couldn't you?'

'Oh, she does,' Terry agreed.

It was true that I felt at home in most places. 'People are always asking me for directions, even if I'm lost.'

'It happened just now, on our way back here from Jaffa,' Terry said. 'A woman with a baby carriage stopped you and wanted the bus stop.'

'If she'd seen how we had to search to find this place earlier,' I said, 'she wouldn't have asked me!'

We both laughed.

'Ah, but it was worth it,' Bero said. 'Wasn't it?'

The knowing look in his eye seemed to carry the suggestion that our coming here fulfilled a destiny.

Surveying the empty lobby, Terry validated his air of mystique. 'Yes, it's very *quiet*,' she said. 'Bero, what do you see for Bobbie?'

He flicked away her words, as if to say *who am I to know?* 'People interest me, that is all.' Nevertheless, he looked at me speculatively.

I didn't like it.

'I think you're very patient and knowledgeable, upright and honest... but wicked.'

I thought he was out of line. 'Thanks!'

'I don't mean evil,' he said. 'I mean bad.'

'I'm not bad!'

'I know what he means,' Terry said. 'You're sparky.'

That much was right. It seemed like I couldn't help losing it.

Just the other day, I got angry when a tourist barged into me in Jerusalem's Old City and kept walking. The Arab storekeeper who overheard and rebuked me for swearing in God's city made me feel ashamed.

At Oasis of Peace, I'd raged at some schoolteachers who'd made the mistake of knocking on our door when rousing their students at 7 am.

And, at our Jerusalem guesthouse, I sang songs from all the American musicals I knew, very loud at 5 a.m., before we left for a bus excursion. This was my revenge on the bunch of American students who'd talked very loud in the corridor outside our room until midnight.

Being furious with Seth had made me furious with the world.

Since I wasn't prepared to admit this man knew my character, I said nothing.

'What do you do for work?' he asked. 'You are a teacher, perhaps?'

'No.'

Terry smiled from Bero to me and back again, like we were all best buddies. 'She had a business but she's retired from that now.'

She was being nice. It had failed. It was a music manufacturing service to the UK record industry that I had founded twenty five years earlier. Its particular strength was manufacturing vinyl records. As vinyl disappeared, online downloads soared and it went under. Years before, Seth had left teaching to help me run it. We ended up at home, drawing down on our private pension fund.

Though I was too young today, at 54, to draw a state pension, the private pension provided a modest income that kept me going.

'Do you like to fish or hunt?' he asked me.

'No.'

I jumped as Terry elbowed me again. 'He knows what's on the rug!' she hissed in my ear.

I hadn't seen the rug. And I most certainly was not going to view this nosy guy's questioning as proof that he was some kind of messenger to us.

'You might enjoy it, if you tried it,' Bero said. 'Do you like to travel?'

'No.'

It was not true, of course. I loved to travel but I wasn't ready to share with him that getting on a flight to Israel had been an act of courage. The risk of blood clots had led me to take aspirin the day before, I wore surgical stockings and drank lots of water during the flight.

'Oh, come on, Bobbie' Terry said. She looked embarrassed by my abruptness.

'I think you'll be travelling,' Bero predicted, his eyes gleaming. 'You'll be taking a trip.'

I pouted. 'I don't do long haul.'

He looked as if he knew better. Then he said, 'Europe. Somewhere like Lake Maggiore.'

'Where's that?' Terry asked.

I filled her in. 'The Italian Lakes.'

'I myself would like to visit Canada,' he told Terry. 'If I came in August, would it still be cold?'

'Oh, no.'

'Are you sure the snow would have melted?'

'Oh, yes.'

'I hate cold.' He hugged himself and shivered.

'It's not cold in Canada in the summer,' she said.

I looked from one to the other, wondering why he was so insistent about the snow melting when, barring a freak storm, there would be none in August. Perhaps he imagined that the whole country was like the North Pole. Or was something else passing between them, some kind of subtext?

Oh, dear. Terry's thinking was rubbing off on me.

'And do you plan to keep the promise you made in Jerusalem?' Bero asked.

Her eyes widened again. 'Yes.'

'Then don't forget your mission,' he said. 'Take care of the fallen birds.'

Now I was totally confused.

4.

We were both exhausted. Agreeing it was time for bed, we said our goodnights to Bero and crossed the lobby to the lift.

'What was the promise you made in Jerusalem?' I whispered in Terry's ear, as we waited.

The doors opened. We stepped inside. The doors closed.

'He knew, Bobbie!' she exclaimed, jumping up and down and making the lift rock. 'He knew all about us. He knew everything that happened today. He must be an angel.'

I was still having a hard time dealing with yesterday's angels. I did not agree Bero was an angel but there would be little point in contradicting her. Experience had shown me that nothing I might say would budge her thinking.

'But the promise?' I repeated at our bedroom door, as I fumbled for the key.

We went in. Decorated in soft shades of peach and lit by wells of lamplight, this room was a last night leap upscale from the simple hostels and guesthouses we had stayed at elsewhere.

'No personal gain,' she said. 'I told you already.'

'Oh, right.'

I was soon lying in my bed with my hands behind my head, wondering about footsteps that turn to the left and to the right, going through ever bigger doors. Though, in my mind's eye, I could clearly picture Terry, weaving her way through arches and entrances and along narrow streets that looked like ancient Israel, it seemed a curious prophecy. As I remembered it, the Hebrew Bible mostly told us to follow God's path and not deviate to the right or the left.

'What about your mission, Terry?' I asked as she emerged from the bathroom.

She pulled back the sheets and got into her bed. 'I've told you everything. All I know is that it's huge.'

Tantalisingly, the rabbi had given no indication of her purpose. 'And thingy downstairs, telling you to take care of the fallen birds?'

'Don't know.'

I wondered if that was me. Was the woman who wanted to become a child a fallen bird?

She lay, propped up by pillows, in the same position as me, hands under her head. She still wore that secret smile. No doubt, she was seeing doors that got bigger as rising glory but it struck me that, equally, they could mean ever greater challenges.

Yawning, I turned on my side. Pretty much all of it was a source of speculation, I decided. The only tangibles, if I discounted the reported prophecies of a person I had never met and the innuendos of the man on reception, were the pictures in Terry's camera and the rug with us on it, if we really were on it.

And the trembling I had felt at King of Kings. That had been real.

'Shall I switch off the light Bobbie?'

'Yeah, thanks,' I murmured, snuggling down.

And Chanelle's inspired suggestion of a cloak to cover me…

'Night,' Terry said.

That had resonated with me because of the cloaks in Ruth's story and my close connection to the Book of Ruth.

'Night night,' I replied.

We had been looking at a carved statue of Ruth when Adam showed up and pointed us to King of Kings. We were coming out of the bookstore with the *Il Rotollo di Rut* book when he appeared again and facilitated Terry's meeting.

It was like a thread was being woven, joining Ruth and her story and my stay in Israel.

5.

I woke up and opened my eyes. The room was still dark but I could make out a heap of sheets at the foot of Terry's bed. She was not in it. I squinted in the direction of the bathroom door. There was no light coming from under it. Where was she?

A ripple, like the flap of a bird's wings, came from down to my left. Terry was on her knees at my bedside. She was praying with her arms thrown wide.

I quickly shut my eyes and pretended to be asleep. But she had spotted me.

'Bobbie, take a pen and write. I know the answer to Chanelle's prayer. You must write this down. I know about the angel in my camera.'

I switched on the light and blinked. The bedside clock read 4 a.m. In just a few hours, Terry would be leaving for the airport and flying home. Filled with a sense of urgency, I reached for my diary. I needed to know what she had to tell me.

She got up off her knees and sat on her bed. Her face was ghostly in the lamplight.

'A lot is happening very fast,' she began. 'Time is running out. You are a large part of this plan. You're going to hunt and you're going to like it. You don't understand right now as you have blinds on your eyes. You see with physical eyes but, soon, you will see through spiritual eyes, of your own volition, not someone else's.'

Everything was still, except my hand, writing frantically, and her husky voice. It seemed to come at me from the shadows of the room, rather than from her mouth. It felt like it had form, like I could touch it.

I was a part of this. I wanted to take a hold of it.

'You need to go to the place told you by the man downstairs...'

'Lake Maggiore?'

'Yes.'

'I don't know when I could get there,' I said.

'Go. Only after that will your next direction for travel be revealed. Don't try to guess it. It's a destination of peace. Don't get stressed about it.'

I was stressed. Her instruction pulled me two ways at once. On the one hand, I was eager to roll up my sleeves and get started. On the other, Terry might just be showing off a delusional prophetic gift and sending me on a wild goose chase.

I was particularly wary of the words 'next direction for travel'. I didn't like the idea of gallivanting around the world. Neither my health nor my budget could stand that.

'Before going on this journey — this will be difficult — you will see your home in a new way upon leaving Israel — there are things in your house holding you back. You need to walk through — don't argue.'

'I'm not,' I said, scribbling to catch up.

'You must release your home of every item holding you back. You cannot go on journeys until you've cleared your house of them.'

I understood very well that she was referring to my tarot cards. Terry saw the beautiful boxed pack that I kept back home in England as a form of witchcraft. On her last visit, she had shut herself up in another room while I read from them.

I liked the way the swirling hair of the characters mingled with cloud-like swirls of colour on the cards, giving them a dreamlike quality. I laid them out in patterns, face down, and turned them over, one by one, trying to work out their meaning.

I couldn't say that I really believed in them. I viewed them rather as a tool to help me imagine a different kind of a life, one where I didn't feel sorry for myself the whole time.

'If you hold back even one item, you will not be able to move forward,' Terry cautioned.

She was right. I should dissociate myself from such things. Though I had never felt a conflict between Judaism and my tarot, there undoubtedly was one. God's word in Deuteronomy 18 was clear: *There shall not be found among you anyone... who interprets omens.*

My future in the cards had never looked very promising, anyway. Over and over, I would turn up the Tower — my world crashing down. As soon as I got home, the cards and books would go out with the rubbish.

Terry pushed back strands of hair that had fallen over her face. 'It will be difficult. You're not used to having a Bridegroom take care of you. You are loved more than you know. You'll begin to feel that more than ever in your life.'

Oh, yes. I really wanted that.

'After you've cleaned out your house, you need to have your house blessed. The person will be brought to you. You won't know but will trust at the right time.'

I had organised a dedication ceremony for my home, when I moved into it, eighteen months before. Family and friends had gathered to read from the Jewish prayer book and nail up a *mezuzah* by the front door. The *mezuzah* was a miniature scroll containing a section from the sixth chapter of the Book of Deuteronomy, rolled up inside a casing. My casing was made of porcelain.

Now Terry was saying that someone would be sent to bless my house again, in the Christian tradition, I supposed. This would happen without my doing anything to initiate it. I couldn't see how that could happen but I wrote it down.

'You need to learn Hebrew, not biblical Hebrew but the Hebrew they speak here.'

'Modern Hebrew?'

'Yes.'

That would be no hardship. I loved foreign languages and had long wanted to learn Hebrew. I'd just never had any reason to do so until now.

'You're an integral part of this,' she finished. 'Have you got it all?'

I finished with a flourish, pleased, with the message she'd given me. 'Yes.'

'Do you have any questions right now?'

My head was swimming with questions, not the least of which was what this was all about. But there seemed little point in asking Terry that. She didn't know herself. 'No'

Even in the midst of uncertainty and mistrust of her prophecies, I felt relief. I felt vindicated. I had told God *hineini* and He hadn't overlooked me or picked my friend instead of me. I was an integral part of this.

I just needed to get my thoughts straight about what this constituted. Most importantly, I needed to work out whether I accepted that a series of supernatural events was unfolding.

'You need to let go,' she said, getting to her feet and coming around the bed. 'There are wonderful things in store for you and many people need you. The time is short. Amen.'

We were a team, in this together. My tears flowed as we hugged.

6.

A breeze, coming off the Mediterranean, blew gently on my face as I sat on the promenade. I would have liked to talk some more with Terry about everything that had happened over the last two days but she was already gone, waving at me through the back window as her taxi set out for the airport at 9.30 this morning.

I felt very alone without her. It was as if my lifeline to Israel had been cut.

I had spent most of the day walking. I had walked right along the seafront and the new marina boardwalk, with its cafes and boutiques, on through *HaYarkon* Park and all the way to the *HaAretz* Museum. There, I had taken pictures of a replica of a biblical home, the type of house Ruth and her mother-in-law, Naomi, might have lived in.

As I walked, I considered spirituality and Israel. I have a deep, emotional connection to this Land that is cherished by Jews the world over, so much so that our Passover meals include the promise to gather, 'Next Year in Jerusalem'. I had come in search of Jewish spirituality to where God claimed the Jews as His people. Yet, prior to Sunday, the only glimpses I had caught of anything resembling spirituality had seemed random.

The most Jewish of these had been a memorable moment in Jerusalem, with the lights of the Old City before me and the night breeze on my face.

There had been nothing Jewish about the times of quiet communion with Terry, as I wrote my journal and she read her Christian book, nor in the glow of pleasure on the face of the Arab chef at Oasis of Peace when he brought us our food...

These flashes had inclined me to think that spirituality couldn't be found in any given place but was grounded in my own response to things external.

My experience at King of Kings on Sunday changed all that. The when and the where of the powerful feeling that overcame me there were of primary importance, for God had chosen to speak into my Jewish heart in a Christian place of worship.

There could be only one explanation for His doing that.

A man was speaking to me. He was about forty years old, dark and handsome. I had no idea how long he had been sitting on the bench beside me.

He repeated his question several times and pointed to his wrist before I understood that he wanted to know the time.

'Ten to four,' I said.

'Thank you.' He coughed.

I returned to my inner world.

Another issue I'd been considering was the significance of the strange photographs that Terry had taken in the place where I was called. If tongues of golden flame the colour of my prayer shawl appeared on my friend's digital display as I trembled, was it beyond belief that they could be a manifestation of what I was experiencing, i.e. the supernatural?

It seemed to me that miracles were often about timing. The Ten Plagues of Egypt may have been naturally occurring phenomena but their supernatural timing spurred Pharaoh to free the Children of Israel. And, if the Red Sea parted at the very moment his chariots bore down on them, wasn't this still a miracle, even if God sent a tsunami?

I bent to take off my sandals.

So what if the pictures were a glitch in Terry's camera? They could still be miraculous. They had certainly led her in the direction of further astonishing discoveries.

The man sitting beside me was walking away. I hadn't noticed him get up. I wondered if perhaps he had wanted to try and strike up a conversation with me, even pick me up.

I was glad he was going. It would have made me very uncomfortable if he'd tried that.

I strolled towards the shallows and kicked up spray. Tomorrow, all this would be wiped from my sight. Tomorrow night, I would sleep in my own bed in my house in England. The prospect neither thrilled nor disheartened me. I was ready to leave.

I was happy in my home but my home did not make me happy.

I sat on a breakwater, dangling my feet to let them dry, and realised with a jolt that home would not be the same now, because I was different. I had been called and claimed. The implications of that, though still unclear, appeared fraught with difficulties.

Running away to a remote cottage or signing up for Voluntary Service Overseas suddenly appeared attractive. If I lived where no one knew me, there would be no need to explain myself and no one would confront or denigrate me.

Someone was blocking out my sunlight.

I squinted up at a man's face. He looked a lot like the guy who'd asked me the time but it wasn't him. The man said something and looked at me expectantly.

'Sorry?'

'Lo medaberet ivrit?'

'No, I don't speak Hebrew,' I confirmed.

He changed to English. 'I said you are the most beautiful woman on this beach.'

'Thank you.' I looked out to sea. He was making me tense. I wished he would go away.

He narrowed his eyes, assessing me. 'What are you, Spanish?'

My dark hair and eyes foiled everyone. I was not about to set him straight.

'What do you want?' I asked, fixing my gaze past his ear at the silhouette of Old Jaffa's fortifications.

He hovered for a moment. 'I guess you're busy.'

I nodded curtly.

I breathed a big sigh of relief as he left.

My silly heart was thudding with fear because I no longer knew how to handle advances that, as a young woman, I would have fielded with ease. The day might have taken a quite different turn if I had been open to chatting with him. We might have walked along the front together, gone for something to eat...

He might have wanted to kiss me. That was a cringe-making thought. I could not imagine being able to respond to anything like that. The prospect of allowing someone to get close was acutely embarrassing and somehow undignified.

Chanelle's prophecy was a million miles from being fulfilled, I thought, as I headed straight back to the hotel.

As I crossed at the crossing, a bunch of young bloods drew up in a beach buggy. Hanging out of their vehicle, they called and wolf whistled at me. They must have been blind. I was old enough to be their mother. Passersby stared as I slunk across, hating the attention.

The shorts that had seemed fine on the beach left me feeling exposed here, in the street.

Bero, on the front desk, grinned as I scooted through the entrance. To me, he looked as much like a predator as any of the men out there. And he had dared to suggest *I* was wicked!

I had told Terry over breakfast that morning that I found him more sleazy than prophetic.

'He was looking into your life and it frightened you,' she chided me gently. 'You've changed from the Bobbie I used to know. You used to challenge the minds of men, now you jump back and accuse them. You strike like a snake at all men.'

I knew this to be true and it saddened me. 'Will I stay like this, Terry?'

'You need to let go.'

'I have no idea how to do that.'

'I think you've a ways ahead of you before you'll trust any man, even Jesus.'

She was probably right. It would take time. But how long?

'Everything's possible,' she added, smiling encouragement. 'We've been sent miracles. And the first Prime Minister of Israel... um...'

'Ben Gurion?'

'Yes. He is supposed to have said that anyone who doesn't believe in miracles in Israel isn't realistic!'

As soon as Bero handed me my key, I bolted up to my room and locked myself in. I spent the evening half-expecting to have to deal with his knock on my door on some trumped-up mission.

It never came.

Chapter 5

1.

'I'll email you a picture of the angel for protection,' Terry said.

We were talking on the phone. She seemed to think I was in danger.

I was sick with pleurisy.

Sharp lung pain kicked in a few days after my return from Israel. My immediate fear was that it was lung clots again. The first time I had them, when I was staying at a writers' retreat in a remote part of Ireland, had been terrifying.

I was admitted to Bantry Cottage Hospital and told to lie still and not move, in case the clots should shift to my heart, which would kill me. My subsequent return to England, with a nurse and oxygen, was a nightmare of anxiety and discomfort.

Pleurisy wasn't half as bad as that. Medication had dealt with the pain. Nevertheless, it had kept me home and pretty much bedbound for twelve days.

I was feeling helpless and sorry for myself. 'That Bero guy asked me whether I liked to travel but I can't, can I? Because this happens.'

'Perhaps he knew your limitations,' Terry replied gently.

'I'm never going to be whizzing across continents.'

I guess I'd wanted to believe I would be.

'We've been sent miracles. Don't forget that.'

I refrained from pointing out that *she* was the one who had been sent miracles. It still rankled that God chose to reveal His signs and wonders to her, when I was the one who was free and available to pursue them.

Fed up with pretty much everything in my life, I thought I'd annoy Terry. 'I've been reading and Christianity is a lot more contentious than I thought.'

'What have you read?'

I had dug out the Christian Bible I used on a university course entitled Christians and Pagans, (when studying for my degree in Social Anthropology and Classical Civilisation).

'All four Gospels and Acts.'

'Wow, that's great!'

'I've had plenty of time.'

Nothing frustrated me more than forced inactivity. My illness had caused me to miss graphic design classes. I hadn't worked on my final major project. I hadn't even downloaded my photos from our trip.

'You've been given an opportunity to go on a journey of discovery.'

'I've done that alright.' I waved my hands about, seeking the right words, even though she couldn't see me. 'Jesus did great stuff. He spoke the truth and healed people. He was a committed Jew.'

'Yes.'

These were the things about Jesus that had impressed me. There were also things I didn't like. 'But, if we're supposed to be meek and turn the other cheek, like he says, how come he was such a political animal? Why did he stir up the masses in Jerusalem against the Pharisees and Sadducees, instead of trying to save them?'

John's Gospel referred to these people as 'the Jews'. Jesus constantly made them look foolish. 'He didn't give them a chance,' I complained.

I was surprised by the depth of emotion hovering just beneath the surface as I said this. I was thinking of Jesus' words. '*I am the way and the truth and the life. No one comes to the Father except through me.*' (John 14:6). This seemed unfair. It gave my own kids no chance.

I wanted to reject this statement but I didn't feel I could argue it with Terry because it was so black and white. I took a different tack. 'Why would we think that Jesus was superior to someone like Gandhi? He led a similar, exemplary life. *He* was very provocative and *he* wound up being assassinated by his own people, just like Jesus.'

'Gandhi never claimed to be the Messiah, or even a prophet,' Terry said.

'Gandhi always thought that, if you expect the best of people, they can't sustain their worst nature. Jesus gave up on the Pharisees. There's other stuff, too. It's in Matthew but it's worse in Luke.'

I reached for the Bible on my bedside table and looked for the page I wanted. 'Here it is, Luke 14, verse 26: *If anyone comes to me and does not hate his father and mother, wife and children, brothers and sisters, yes, and his own life also, he cannot be my disciple.*'

'Yes?'

'Well, that's terrible. I can't hate my family.'

I was confused. This instruction flew in the face of all kinds of commandments from the Hebrew Bible, including the one to honour your father and your mother, which was one of the Ten Commandments. Yet Jesus said that he came to fulfil *Torah*, not abolish it.

I wondered why I was getting so worked up about this. Was I really getting stuck on the small print or sick and gunning for an argument? Or was it that I was looking for a way out?

Terry's quiet response surprised me. 'Scripture's hard when you read through secular eyes. Try reading it with spiritual eyes.'

I didn't know what to say to that.

'Read it again, Bobbie, with spiritual eyes.'

Perhaps I would. Meanwhile, I had a further question. 'I was thinking about the rug. I found horses in Revelation...'

'Revelation's a hard book.'

'Was the author on LSD?'

I thought the crackling on the line would go on forever. When, eventually, she spoke her voice was gentle. 'I see your sickness as time out of time, Bobbie. God wanted you to read the New Testament. He knows you don't do rest unless He makes you. That's why you're sick.'

The idea that this frustrating downtime could be a demonstration of God's love for me was something new. It made me smile.

'Take comfort in the fact that they're praying for us in Israel, for both of us,' Terry said.

A congregation of strangers, praying for me, seemed weird.

At synagogue, you come in, take your place, stand up and sit down, as directed by the rabbi on the dais. The prayers are formal, read from a prayer book, even those for healing or for the dead. At the end of the service, you make *Kiddush*: the rabbi gives thanks for wine, then bread and everybody has some. After that, the conversation is about secular things.

If being prayed for by Christians was like Chanelle's prayers for me, I wanted that very much.

And then Terry began to pray for me, down the phone line. 'Dear Lord, please bless Bobbie. Keep her, encourage her. Bestow your abundant love upon my friend. She is of great value and I know Your love for her is great.

'Open her eyes, heart, spirit, body and mind to Your Kingdom and its beauty. Give her answers to the many questions she has that trouble her. Take away the burden from her chest. Cause her to be as light as a feather.

'Introduce Yourself to her in such a way that she will know

beyond a shadow of a doubt that You are who You said You are and You behaved the way You did in the passages she is reading for good reason.

'Minister to her. Cause the Holy Spirit to come to her. Open her spiritual eyes and give her clarity. Purify the space where she lives and heal her body. Protect us both. Thank you, Lord.'

Her beautiful words brought tears to my eyes. Now I knew that I loved being prayed for.

I said, 'Amen.'

2.

After our conversation, I leaned back against the pillows and closed my eyes. Gradually, a picture formed in my mind's eye of a big, red stone — a ruby. I imagined it tilting this way and that so that I could see its depths and glowing embers, shot with flames.

I didn't understand this beautiful picture but it made me feel so much better. Aggression left me and I began to believe that soon I would be well again.

Ruby was my late mother's name. Though she had died sixteen years before, I still missed her. I still would find myself hovering by the phone, longing to pick it up and pour out my life to her. Like the Woman of Proverbs 31, whose worth is far above rubies, my mother was a good woman, diligent, wise and kind.

I wondered whether the ruby came to me as a result of Terry's loving prayer. The timing of its appearance seemed appropriate: right now, she was nurturing me like a mother.

I searched online for red rubies, when I was well enough to sit at my computer again. I quickly found a rich, Burmese stone that resembled the ruby of my vision. It was being offered direct from the jeweller in — well, here was a surprise — Ramat Gan, Israel.

The guide on our excursion to Nazareth and Capernaum had explained how Israel became a centre of excellence for cutting diamonds and other gemstones: Jewish jewellers from Europe had settled there in large numbers, after the Second World War. The country was now world-renowned for its gem cutting.

Gazing upon the myriad lights and darks of this ruby was like unwrapping a gift I had always wanted and never knew it. I wondered whether I was meant to buy this stone but soon rejected the idea. Buying myself expensive jewellery would only underscore my state of woman alone, I felt.

Terry was excited to hear about my vision of a ruby from Israel.

'Perhaps it represents the blood,' she suggested.

I didn't know what she meant.

'You see, the blood washes you clean.'

I winced as images from the shower stabbing scene in the movie *Psycho* sprang to mind. 'Clean from what?'

'From sin.'

'Yes,' I said, getting her meaning. 'Temple sacrifices.'

I explained that the leprous house from my *Bat Mitzvah Torah* portion was sprinkled with the blood of a sacrificed pigeon, to cleanse it.

'The house could become unclean again,' she said. 'Jesus' blood spilled on the cross made us white as snow, once and for all.'

This sounded like Christian rhetoric to me. I knew I wasn't perfect — I was ready to repent for all the bad things I did by apologising to God on *Yom Kippur*, the Jewish Day of Atonement, and fasting — but I saw myself as a fundamentally good person, not a sinner.

Suddenly, she switched subject. 'Listen, Bobbie, I have news! Israel called!'

'Israel?'

'Members of the congregation praying for us. Yonaton. They took my address. They want to send me something. I think it's the rug!'

This was exciting news indeed. She could send me pictures. I'd actually get to see it.

Wow. For me, a vision of a beautiful ruby, cut in Israel, for Terry a rug. It seemed Israel had followed us both home.

3.

My friend, Veronica, sipped the coffee I had made her. 'There is a wonderful quiet calm and joy in coming to God,' she said.

She was a Jew who believed in Jesus and the one person I felt able to tell about what happened to me in Israel.

I wasn't feeling quiet calm and joy right now, not at all.

Outside, the garden fence was swaying in the gusting wind. I knew how it felt. My heart was saying, 'accept Jesus', because I believed in the signs and wonders, because it felt right, because to do so would be emotionally uplifting.

And because I wanted desperately to be 'an integral part of this'.

However, my head was still refusing to trust what my heart was telling it. I wasn't ready to admit that my Jewish faith was incomplete, not to say flawed, and I was unwilling to see myself as a needy person, someone who, potentially, might clutch at straws.

I was afraid of all the sweeping changes in my life that crossing over to Christianity would set in motion.

I needed to talk things through with a Jewish believer and Veronica was the only one I knew. She was well-known for her annoying evangelising amongst the South London Jewish community. The Jews, who don't evangelise but look inward and keep their beliefs to themselves, would stonewall her.

Though I had invited her here today, I was concerned that she might seek to chalk me up as someone she'd won over with her message. Her aim seemed to be to open our eyes to something she'd found but we were all too blind to see.

I ran my fingers through hair left lank by pleurisy, and hesitantly handed her the ammunition she needed to turn me into a trophy. 'I felt Him in the Prayer Tower in Jerusalem, when Chanelle prayed Psalm 37 over me.'

She opened her bible and read the psalm out loud.

It was beautiful. But one line bothered me. 'That bit about dwelling in the Land...'

Her olive green eyes opened wide. 'That means the Kingdom of God.'

Though I had no understanding what the Kingdom of God was, I let out a sigh of relief. Terry had told me to learn modern Hebrew and had hinted I would be returning to Israel on God's work. 'I thought it meant Israel. I thought it was telling me I was supposed to live there.'

The idea of being alone in Israel didn't appeal to me at all.

She took my hand and held it between her own. 'Don't try to second guess God. His purpose will unfold. Be patient and pray.'

'But sometimes God sends us where we don't want to go. Look at Jonah. When he resisted the instruction to prophesy in Ninevah, he ended up in the belly of a whale!'

Though she laughed, her usual seriousness quickly returned. 'Many people pursue only their own happiness,' she said. 'But self-gratification is a shallow reward. To achieve true happiness, we must be obedient.'

Though the weather today was wet and grey, here inside was cosy. As the gas log fire's flames danced, I told her about Chanelle's amazing prayer for me. 'She asked God to take me as His obedient bride and give me rest, until such time as He should provide a new husband for me.'

Veronica's golden locks shook like spaniel's ears. 'You have a husband.'

A familiar, tight ball of self-pity clogged my throat.

She had not given up on the idea of reconciliation, had even been to see Seth the previous year, to try and talk him round. He had told her we parted because I became too dissatisfied with him, which had seemed a curious sort of analysis. Surely, the issue for anyone who cared would have been why?

'Adultery is the only acceptable grounds for divorce,' Veronica said.

I assumed this was her Christian belief because Jews were permitted to divorce.

Though our grounds were mutual consent, Seth had been adulterous. 'When he wanted someone, it was someone else.'

'He took a mistress *after* you left,' she pointed out.

Though this was true, I felt she was being unduly harsh in the face of my fragility.

'Mistresses,' I corrected. I resented her implication that his dalliances were acceptable.

I had left as a result of what a lawyer friend had called, 'constructive dismissal.' After my years of illness and the failure of our business, Seth got so busy with his hobbies that I was pretty much excluded from his life.

The late Princess Diana famously said that there were three of them in her marriage to Prince Charles and it was a bit crowded. I was all alone in mine and it was a lot lonely.

He never came after me. He didn't call. He made no attempt to save the marriage. Resentment festered and it broke my heart that our thirty plus years together meant nothing to him. I had thought we were for life and had never expected it to end like this.

Any lingering hopes of reconciliation I might have harboured were shattered when I learned that he was seeing someone, just a few months after we separated. Hoping against hope that it was untrue, I phoned and tackled him about this final nail in the coffin of our relationship. He admitted to having a girlfriend and even volunteered that she was not the first. 'A person needs some kisses and cuddles,' he explained.

My insides churned. I needed some kisses and cuddles.

Joining a Ceroc jive class had been one of our last-ditch attempts at trying to enjoy one another's company. We had always loved to dance together. But I didn't like the class. I wanted to dance with him, not change partners every few minutes, or stand out and watch, as I often had to, because there were more women than men.

He liked it, however, and kept on going alone, after I stopped, with the opposite result to what I wanted: he was out, doing his own thing, even more than before.

And, at the next party we went to, I found he had learned new steps I couldn't follow. Because of the Ceroc, the one thing we had left, the dancing together that I loved, was gone.

I blew my nose. Veronica was nodding. 'Men are not like us. They have needs.'

'I have needs!' I flared.

'Marriage is for life.' Her voice was gentle, her tone firm. 'Your duty was to stay.'

I'd asked her to come to discuss what happened in Israel, not so that she could lecture me about my failed marriage. Her stance seemed to be that things would be required of me as a Christian that weren't required before.

She opened her bible again. 'Look here at Matthew 19. Jesus says that the only acceptable grounds for divorce is sexual immorality. Seth was faithful within the marriage, wasn't he, Bobbie?'

I didn't want to do this anymore.

'A man who wants to keep doors open doesn't take a mistress.' I gathered up our empty coffee mugs and took them to the kitchen. 'Jewish Law allows divorce.'

I wanted her to go so I could have a good cry but she wasn't done with me yet. 'That person in the Prayer Tower was wrong. You won't be able to remarry. Anyone who divorces, except for sexual immorality, and remarries commits adultery.'

'Don't tell me Christ stopped people escaping from an abusive marriage.'

'Seth wasn't abusive.'

'You don't have to use your fists to be an abuser.'

4.

A few days after Veronica's visit, I finally sat at my computer with a mug of hot tea to download all the many photos I took during my trip. It was almost a month since my return from Israel,

I couldn't think of a better way to spend a rainy April Saturday afternoon than to relive those colourful moments.

Here was the view across the vineyards to the chapel with the clanging bell below the Oasis of Peace Centre, here the turquoise waters of the Dead Sea backed by the mauve mountains of Moab that Ruth and Naomi would have descended. Here was the strange picture of the Ruth statue in the antiques store, with Adam's white cab superimposed over it. And the peaceful Garden Tomb that Terry took me to.

As I cropped and saved, one picture in particular caught my attention. It was taken on our last Saturday, the day before King of Kings. We were on the coach back to Jerusalem from the Galilee excursion. As we drove along the Jordan River Valley, I'd pointed my camera past Terry and clicked at the china blue sky, framed by fluffy clouds. I couldn't remember why.

Frowning, I leaned into my computer screen and screwed up my eyes. There certainly seemed to be something unexpected about the result. In the sky, silhouetted in a deeper blue than it was what looked like a man, with arms outstretched.

I went and switched on the overhead light and came back to look again. I clicked 'print' and waited for a better look.

As the printer rattled into its 'Oh, my lumbago' routine, two teenage girls appeared in the street outside my window. As they walked, they swung the High Street fashion store bags that contained their purchases. They were unaware of me, watching from behind the slatted wooden blind. The clouds overhead were turning charcoal. We were in for more rain, for sure.

I took the printout in my hands and was so excited that I felt like shouting out to them to come see what I had.

What I had thought I was seeing was really there. Across the sky above the Jordan, was a man in the sky. His arms were extended, like Christ on the Cross. But there was no suffering in him. His welcoming arms put me in mind of pictures I'd seen of the Jesus carving on top of the Sugarloaf Mountain in Rio de Janeiro, Brazil.

I hadn't realised that something special was happening, any more than Terry did as she snapped her angel pictures at King of Kings. It was uplifting to think that, invisible to me, the sky had been filled with God, waiting to embrace me and welcome me home, like the Daddy of the Prodigal Son.

The strangeness of the picture could, no doubt, be explained away as an effect of light through the window of the bus or a camera quirk. That didn't detract from the miracle: the timing of its message was perfect and exactly what I craved.

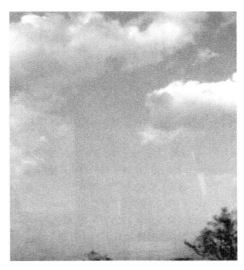

Not only did it reach out to me to tell me I was wanted, it also transformed how I saw my role in the adventure I felt I was embarking upon. Taken the day *before* Terry's angel pictures, it promoted me from camp follower to first called.

Jesus chose me and was there, with his arms open to me, even before I met Him. It was beautiful.

I pushed back my stool and raised my hands, crying, 'Thank You, Lord!' As I did so, the heavens opened and arrows of living water fell from the sky.

5.

Although, by now, I had given a lot of consideration to the beautiful faith I was drawn to, I told myself I was still only window-shopping. I decided to visit a Christian church, to see what I could see.

Veronica said she might be able to meet me at her church, providing her husband, who didn't approve of her faith, went out to play golf. I turned her down. I wasn't ready to be introduced to a lot of people. I preferred to go somewhere alone. Then, if I felt uncomfortable, I could slip out quietly.

I had no preconceived ideas about denomination. The church nearest to home happened to be Pentecostal.

I walked up and down outside before going in briskly, hoping no Jews I knew would see me. I was a familiar face to most of the South London Jewish community and had attended Sabbath worship at my local synagogue just the day before.

The service had already started. As I slipped into a pew, I immediately found the drumbeat compelling and the singing rousing. The prayers were heartfelt and inspirational. In no time at all, I found I was trembling, exactly like at King of Kings.

I was overjoyed to realise that had not been a one-off and I could connect with this exquisite feeling of excitement, interwoven with deep, relaxing peace, again. I closed my eyes and thanked God for the balm and blessing of worship.

Everyone sat down and the preacher, a charismatic speaker, explained that it is our human nature to sin. He gave examples of how even toddlers can be violent tricksters and tellers of tall stories.

I was grateful for this sermon which clarified the meaning of the term 'original sin' for me. This sermon brought home the value and significance of Jesus' washing away our sins through his sacrifice on the cross.

Now I understood what Terry had meant about the cleansing power of Jesus' blood, spilled on the cross. How lovely it would be if the vision I had been given of a ruby symbolised the precious blood of Jesus that had the power to wash me white as snow.

The pastor said that a fresh start and a clean slate, is offered to everyone. 'Anyone who has not yet done so but feels ready to make a commitment to Jesus, please raise your hand.'

My hand wanted to go up but I was terrified of the flood gates I would open by raising it. Neither did I want to draw attention to myself.

You might think that it would have been easier for me to remain as I was, with my head down. Not so. A voice inside my head was shouting: *Put your hand up!* and tugging at my arm. I had no choice but to obey.

Gingerly, I raised my hand.

The pastor said to wait at the end of the service. As people left, I remained seated and, after a moment, a woman of about fifty came up to me. She was tall and business-like, with black-rimmed glasses and a clipboard. She told me her name and asked me for my contact details.

Still feeling dazed and otherworldly, I gave her the information.

'I want to speak to the pastor,' I said. I wanted to ask him about the signs and wonders.

'He doesn't do that.'

'But I need to speak to him.'

'He doesn't see women alone. I'm sure you can understand why. You can speak to me.'

I didn't see why I should have to speak to her when it was the pastor who had inspired me. I didn't even know what her role was here. And I hadn't said I wanted to see the pastor *alone*.

At that moment, he walked by us. I grabbed the opportunity to intercept him. 'I was moved by your message this morning. I'd like an appointment to see you.'

'I told her you don't do that,' the woman interjected.

'I don't do that,' he said and kept walking.

Tears welled up. I looked at the floor. 'I think I've made a mistake.'

She spoke a little more gently. 'As I said, I can speak to you.'

I brushed her words away with my hand and teetered out into the drumming traffic like a drunkard. Inexplicably, what I felt was ashamed.

6.

'Right messages, wrong people,' Terry concluded, when I phoned that evening to tell her of my confusion, disappointment and festering resentment.

I was surprised when she told me that she, too, had met with rejection in a church that day.

'When the people in Israel called, they prophesied that bad men would come against me,' she said. 'I never imagined it would happen in a church.'

She had attended a white plank, New England style church in a town near her home. After the singing, the pastor called forward a handful of students who were graduating as missionaries. Extending his arms towards them, he asked for God's blessing on their various missions.

'Thank you, Jesus,' Terry whispered, taking this commission as referring to herself and the mission prophesied to her in Israel.

The pastor continued, 'Watch over them, be with them in all their endeavours and keep them. Some of them will feel strange in distant lands. Help them to feel right at home. They will be in a place that corresponds to their talents and Your calling. Bless their work with success.'

Terry was on her feet, swaying. Her teeth began to chatter. She let out a groan.

Heads turned around to look at her.

She clasped her hands to heaven. 'Yes. Oh please, Jesus, yes. Thank you.'

'Some will face danger.'

'Keep me safe, Jesus, I pray.'

'This is not the place for this kind of display,' hissed a woman, sitting along the pew from her.

It made me smile to picture Terry, all emotion, in a church full of silent, stoic people. I imagined their discomfort and knew, if I'd been there with her, I'd have blushed.

Nothing, it seemed, could make Terry blush. She reached out and grasped the woman's hand. 'Can't you feel the power coursing through me?'

The poor woman yanked her hand away. 'You're disrupting the service.'

The pastor invited the congregation to pray for the missionaries and donate what they could to help fund them.

Tears streamed down Terry's face. 'Oh, thank You, Jesus! I love you.'

An usher approached. He asked her to leave but she carried on in similar fashion, ignoring him.

A second usher came to back up the first one up. 'You can't pray like that here.'

'This is not of God,' the woman along the pew said. 'The Holy Spirit wouldn't do this during the service.'

These words made me switch from grinning about Terry to wholeheartedly supporting her. I didn't like the ushers or the sanctimonious woman with her rules about what the Holy Spirit would or wouldn't do.

I was pretty sure it was the Holy Spirit that had got a hold of me that morning and made me look tipsy.

A man sitting in front of Terry wheeled around. 'For God's sake, get out of this church!'

She staggered back, wide-eyed. 'Can't you feel the anointing?'

Three ushers bundled her into a side room, probably the vestry. One of them suggested that the Jewish Star of David hanging from her neck was a satanic symbol.

When the service finished, the pastor came in.

Terry said, 'Your words today were a true blessing,'

'I've seen this kind of thing before,' the usher told him. 'She has a demon. You should take her away and deliver her.'

He turned and left the room.

'That's amazing,' I told her. 'Our lives are running along parallel paths. We were both rejected on the same day, by pastors on two different continents.'

'I know that these are good people, in their heart of hearts,' Terry told me sadly. 'But they believe that prayers only come from the front of the church and that the Holy Spirit only works at the front.'

She was right, although I felt there was an issue of her own lack of restraint that she wasn't addressing. I'd recently read in 1 Peter that we were to *show proper respect* to others and *love the family of believers*. Surely that included not upstaging the pastor or stealing the missionaries' moment?

7.

I pored over the pictures of the rug that Terry emailed me, as soon as she received it. The rug was a beautiful article, unmistakably Persian.

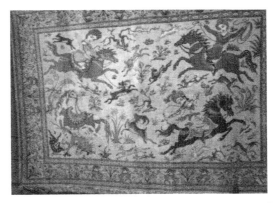

It was uncanny how the weaver had caught my quirks and traits. I never expected the likeness of me to be so accurate.

My eyes were big and dark, my nose straight, my mouth wonky. I had a narrow chin and wide hips, an English pear. Left-handed, I held a rope in my left hand. My eyebrows were characteristically knit together in concentration as I pursued a leaping ibex on a fiery Arabian chestnut.

The ibex looked identical to the one that sprang in front of the car as I drove with Terry beside the Dead Sea. In one graceful leap, it had covered the width of the road and launched itself up the mountain face.

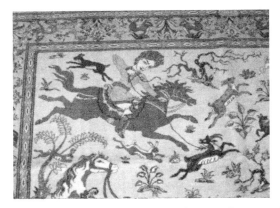

Terry's horse was blue-grey. She faced front, lasso in hand and arms spread wide in typical, expansive gesture. She looked exactly like her little, stick of dynamite self as we galloped towards one another, long manes and tails flying.

Filled with excitement, I picked up the phone and called her. 'What about this, then?'

'I know,' she said. 'It's unbelievable.'

'It's gorgeous.'

'It comes from Iran and it was woven in 1952.'

I was born in 1952. 'How do you know that?'

'Yonaton gave me all the background info,' she said. 'He called at the exact same time it was delivered.'

It was unnerving to think that someone in Iran was weaving a rug bearing my adult likeness as I was being born in England.

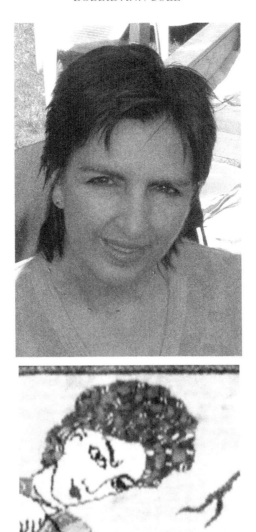

'It was the worst possible time,' Terry continued. 'Don's men have been here all week, working in the sawmill.'

Her husband built log homes for a living. He had a sawmill next door to the house.

'They were taking their morning break in my kitchen. They made a lot of dumb suggestions about what I did in Jerusalem to make someone send me a rug. I ignored them and sat on the floor to undo the wrappings. Oh, the scent that came wafting out at me, Bobbie! It took me straight back to Jerusalem.'

'Yes,' I said, picturing a labyrinth of narrow streets. 'The exotic foods and spices of the *souk*, the heady perfumes.'

'No, the musty warehouse where God made me His girl!'

My laughter was piqued with sadness. I should have been there with her.

'What do you think about the border?' she asked.

I hadn't got as far as looking at that yet. 'What about it?'

'Deer and rabbits.' Her tone was smug.

I took a look. 'Oh, yes and flowers. It's lovely.'

'Yonaton saw the deer and rabbits around my house,' she reminded me.

'Don't rub it in.'

'And Bero asked me about them. I think he's one of the men on the rug.'

There were four riders in all. I was in the top left corner, Terry the right. The other two were moustached men, not Westerners like us but Middle Eastern-looking.

I peered at my computer screen. Neither one of them looked like Bero to me.

The man immediately below me, in the bottom left corner, was off his horse and down on one knee. A knife was in his hand, poised to skin a felled deer that had an arrow sticking out of its back. His horse, a spotted appaloosa, stood behind him, looking wistfully back into the picture.

The other man, below Terry and diagonally opposite me, was wielding a bow and arrow as he galloped off stage on a black horse.

'Well, I'm dying of curiosity.'

'I want you to find out everything you can about this rug, Bobbie.'

I promised I'd certainly try.

She returned to her account of the rug's arrival. 'Lonnie saw the delivery truck pull up outside the house and came running in from the barn. He stared at the rug, with his hands on his hips, like the men. Then he pointed his finger: *Dat's you, Mom!*'

This was no surprise.

Terry put on her man voice. '*Reckon he'd be 'bout right wi'that*, the men all agreed. Then Don pointed at you and said: *And that's your friend.*'

'But I've never even met your husband!'

'He recognised you from my photos of Israel,' she said.

'Unbelievable.' It must *really* look like me.

'As all this was going on, the phone rang. Yonaton was calling to see if the rug had arrived safely. I was jumping up and down and saying: *It's wonderful!*'

'It certainly is,' I agreed. It was more than wonderful. It was totally awesome.

As far as I was concerned, this old Persian rug was God's confirmation that He had a mission in mind for me. A mission was everything that I wanted and had asked Him to send. Here was my purpose, the answer to my *hineini*.

If I could only figure out what it all meant.

8.

A few weeks later, a Sunday evening service in a tent in a park gave me the final nudge I needed to commit. The tent was an outreach, jointly hosted by Veronica's Church of England congregation and the local Baptist Church. She said she might be able to get away to join me but didn't show.

A man who was clearly simple went up to speak at the open mic. He delighted in the landmarks of the outreach as he saw them and closed by saying, 'I know that the angels are looking down on us from above tonight.'

I looked around at everyone smiling and applauding and I felt included in the warmth radiating from them, even though they were strangers to me. Perhaps the simple man was right.

He sat down and another man came forward. Clearly this man had been involved in the organisation of the outreach for he thanked everyone for their hard work and pointed out that all members of the Body of Christ, however humble their tasks, had equally important roles.

'It may not be given to all of us to see a burning bush or follow a pillar of flame,' he said, 'but we all share in the Kingdom.'

His words made me sit up and listen. I had seen such signs and wonders, but was still dithering.

At that moment, I knew I should dither no more.

Back home, I took some quiet time in my bedroom. Though the lights were off, it wasn't really dark. Amber from the streetlight pierced the venetians, casting stripes across the foot of my bed.

In Judaism, it was just not done to go down on your knees. This was probably because it was what Christians did.

Tonight, I wanted to be a Christian. I knelt down and put my palms together.

I had never been one for making much of personal prayer — God and I had always been more on chatting terms. I usually tuned in when I wanted to talk through a problem or was in the throes of some kind of crisis.

Tonight, I wanted to confess my sins and ask God for forgiveness. It was difficult to begin but, once I started, I couldn't stop. It took a lot longer than I expected.

There was much to say about my temper, my selfishness, the injustices I had perpetrated and the lies I had told. There was much to regret about hurting people and my uncaring attitude. There had been chivvying and bullying of my children, downright grumpiness, self-righteousness and self-pity. There had been a lot of kidding myself.

I had failed to do many things I might have done and done things I wished I hadn't.

I went on and on.

By the time I was done, the tears were falling. I felt so blessed, so grateful. I thanked God for Jesus in my life. I thanked Him for forgiveness. And I asked:

God, please send me what I need. Open my eyes to what is. Don't make me a lamb bleating after the flock or a desperate person who clings to any buoy in a choppy sea. Make me someone who walks barefoot in the desert, upright, unaffected by the heat, focused upon the rhythm of the walk. And let the sun warm my flesh as I stretch my hands towards You.

Chapter 6

1.

How to interpret the rug was an enigma that was constantly in my thoughts.

The rug's background was the same buttery gold colour as both my *Bat Mitzvah* prayer shawl and Terry's angel photos. I didn't know what that signified, if anything, but I liked that the three were linked. The repetition of this colour gave me a sense of sequence, of progression towards something.

Terry and I discussed endlessly whether the hunting scene was a metaphor for something else.

'I will be heralding and you will be the one doing the catching,' she said. 'You're the roper.'

I looked again at my computer screen and the pictures she had sent me. Her spread arms and forward-facing pose gave her the appearance of announcer, whereas I wore a frown of concentration as I tried to rope the ibex. Our tasks were well-suited to our personalities.

Terry was convinced that this represented the two of us evangelising but I had no reason, beyond her assertion, to accept this.

'I've found out quite a bit about traditional, Iranian story rugs,' I told her. 'It's unusual that the women should look Western.'

'They look exactly like the two of us,' she riposted. 'That's even more unusual.'

'Well, yes,' I agreed. 'They're woven by tent-dwelling tribes who probably lived out their lives without ever seeing a Western woman. Especially if our rug was made back in 1952, as you were told. Different tribes evolved distinctive styles but I've not come across anything that looks like ours.'

The rugs I'd seen in the Victoria and Albert Museum and fancy Knightsbridge shop windows, or viewed online at the Carpet Museum of Iran, lacked the vibrant life of ours. Their characters seemed two-dimensional and unrealistic, by comparison, with static, stylised people and horses, looking on at the action.

'The composition of our rug is also odd,' I went on. 'Both men are facing outwards, off the rug, but we...'

'... look like we're on a collision course,' she finished for me.

I laughed. 'Yes, why is that?'

'I don't know, Bobbie. Not yet.'

'And what we're doing on the rug looks more like ranching than hunting,' I said. 'But the sequence of events makes no...' A sudden realisation hit me so hard that I slapped my own forehead. 'Oh, my goodness! Of course!'

'What?'

'It's a story rug, right? We've been reading it left to right, like an English book, but that's the wrong way. Oooh!' I tried to scoop my typing school in for an even closer look at my monitor, the front wheels left the ground and I almost fell backwards. 'We need to read it from right to left, like Hebrew or Arabic.'

I was triumphant. This felt like a major breakthrough.

'Yes!' she cried. 'So...?'

I tried to piece the story together. 'You're in the top right hand corner so, chronologically, you go first. You send the prey my way, like a beater, and I try to catch it, top left.'

'The ibex?'

'Yes. Next is the man on the black horse occupying the bottom right of the picture. He's about to shoot another ibex with his bow and arrow and gallop away.'

'...And last comes Number Four, bottom left,' she said. 'He's going to skin the deer that has the arrow in its back. I've noticed he has richer clothing than our turbans and tunics. He's wearing an embroidered robe and a crown-like headdress.'

She was right. But the information didn't seem to take us anywhere helpful.

'The events escalate as you follow the story,' I said, trying to sum up the action. 'We go from you, waving your arms full of joy, to... a death.'

I found this conclusion puzzling as well as disappointing.

'One man is Bero and the other Yonaton,' she maintained.

Since I didn't really remember what either of them looked like, I had no reason to contradict her. But I had no reason to agree with her, either. 'You think?'

One thing I had noticed I wasn't going to mention to her was that Number Four had a little cleft chin, exactly like Seth.

I didn't want him on the rug.

'Why the switch from ibex to deer at the end?' Terry wondered.

'What can that mean?'

'The deer is dead but the ibex lives on...' My voice tailed away. There seemed more questions now than when we'd started out. I was at a loss how to go on. 'Oh, I don't know.'

It was frustrating but, as far as the rug was concerned, I would have to wait for revelation.

2.

It was lunchtime on a late June day. I was sitting alone at a garden table out front of a local eighteenth century coaching inn that, inside, had received a cool, contemporary makeover. The sun was playing hide and seek with the clouds.

I was waiting for Seth, of all people.

I wasn't looking forward to this meeting but I was hoping it would help me summon up forgiveness. Forgiveness was the word on everyone's lips and something the seven-week course I was taking in Divorce and Separation Recovery advocated.

Not forgiving was holding me prisoner in an angry place, looking backward, unable to move forward. Tears of frustration could still catch me unawares, especially in the bathroom. There wasn't much to distract me, sitting on the loo: sometimes, I would crumple and bawl.

He was coming towards me now.

I really wasn't looking forward to this.

We exchanged half smiles and an awkward peck on the cheek. I stole a sideways glance as we went inside. His olive eyes held none of their former warmth. I was already disappointed.

My difficulty was that every scenario of forgiveness I played out included him asking for it.

It wasn't going to happen.

If it did, would I have to forgive him and take him back?

'Here's a table,' Seth said.

I didn't like his choice. It was gloomy here, at the back of the restaurant. Three young guys were lounging and laughing nearby.

'I saw a nice table out front,' I suggested. It was high like this one, with strips of summer sunlight flickering across it. And it was away from these young bloods.

He sat at the dark table as if I hadn't spoken.

So, he wasn't feeling conciliatory or he'd have listened to my wishes.

I clambered up beside him and stole another sideways glance. He was still a handsome man, his body was still athletic, but he had lost some hair. It had turned silver.

Despite the way he had talked to me as if I were tiresome when I called, I'd gathered from Tania, who was home from university for the summer, that he wanted us to get back together. Though I could see no way back, I felt duty-bound to explore the possibilities. I didn't want to turn out the baddie in this story.

Soon, the guys next to us were swearing and being saucy with the waitress. Seth looked sheepish. He knew he'd got it wrong. 'We'll move.'

The table I had suggested was now taken. We sat where we could, along the wall.

As we scanned the menu, I talked to him about Holy Trinity Brompton Church, which ran the Divorce and Separation Recovery Course. This Church in South Kensington was also the home of the world-renowned Alpha Course, which he'd never heard of. 'I've started attending every Sunday.'

I found the worship there dynamic and charismatic.

'And I'm going to join one of their pastorate groups,' I said. 'They have them all over London.'

Seth seemed to be listening. Despite my misgivings about him, I saw a chink of light. I imagined him praising Jesus at HTB with me. One of the lovely aspects of services there was the way couples worshipped together. Men would lay protective arms across their women's shoulders.

I began to tell him about my new faith in Jesus.

He soon doused my enthusiasm. 'That imposter!' he cut in.

My eyebrows shot up. He always was opinionated and tactless but such behaviour in the present context also made it very clear he wasn't looking to woo me.

'What makes you so sure?' I asked.

He didn't seem to know much about Jesus and thought He featured in the Jewish Bible but had been rejected by the rabbis.

I grinned at the truth in that. The *Tanach was* full of references to the Messiah that the rabbis overlooked.

'Is this HTB some kind of a cult?' he wanted to know.

'It's Church of England,' I retorted.

This wasn't the first time it had been suggested that I'd joined some strange sect. Other family members, particularly my three kids, were whispering behind the scenes. It was plain ridiculous.

We got on to the subject of discerning God's will. He didn't agree with me when I said, 'I believe God is in control.'

'I believe we can control our lives.'

'We can't control the next minute!'

'I think we should move away from the subject of religion,' he said.

I agreed.

The waitress came and I ordered a salmon salad. He ordered roast beef, baked potatoes with Yorkshire pudding and a bottle of wine.

'I love my tennis,' he said, as soon as she left us.

This felt like lunch with a colleague. There was no love, or even lust, in him. I suspected that my own eyes were empty, too. Around him, I was guarded.

'I know.'

'I hang-out at the club with my friends after playing, sometimes until 10 pm.'

I didn't know why he'd brought this up or where he was going with it, so I just kept the pot boiling. 'You used to play weekend afternoons.'

'Still do.' He grinned. 'And I like my dancing.'

Ouch. I hated the Ceroc jive classes that, at the end of our marriage, had left me at home while he went out to dance with lots of different women.

I could not resist a snipe. 'Was that where you met your girlfriend?'

'Which one?' He started to grin but then changed his mind and tried for a serious look. 'I'd give her up, if we got back together.'

'Oh that's all right, then,' I said sweetly. 'But not the dancing?'

'No.'

It hit me that he was negotiating, angling to keep the post-tennis drinks and the Ceroc.

I wondered why he would try to get back together, if he didn't want to spend time with me. Was it so I could clean the house and cook his supper?

Maybe he didn't want to look like the baddie himself.

Veronica had said Jesus wanted this, Tania had accused me of pushing her Dad away and my course leaders had made it very clear that reconciliation was the best possible outcome.

But it was looking like a recipe for more hurt. We couldn't even get on.

'Why did you turn away from me, Seth?'

He stared across the room, seemingly deep in thought. Eventually, he said, tight-lipped, 'You always have to spoil it.'

'I have to know.'

The waitress set a bottle of red wine on the table and he filled our glasses. He took a sip. I followed suit.

He looked uncomfortable. 'I think I took you for granted.'

It didn't make any sense. 'How can you take a person for granted who's just nearly died on you?'

A dear friend, Valerie, had suggested that Seth put up a shield when I was sick. Convincing himself he didn't care protected him from getting hurt, she thought. It was a comforting idea, one that allowed for love, underneath the neglect.

Real or assumed, the neglect looked the same. It was what pushed me out the door.

Our food arrived. I had started saying grace before meals but decided it would be best to skip that here and avoid any more trouble. I thanked God for the food in my head and asked for the gift of forgiveness, as He had forgiven me.

My salmon was cooked to perfection but I pushed my food around the plate. I was still brim-full of hurt and resentment. 'I was a good wife. You never gave me any credit for the things I did.'

'You were always trying to compete with me.' He punctuated his words with a flourish of his fork. His tone implied he was stating the obvious.

But it wasn't. This was something totally new that I'd never heard him say before.

How could he believe I was competing with him? I had always tried to be a loving and industrious wife, like the good woman of Proverbs 31.

I remembered, years before, Seth told me a client had asked: *So what's it like being married to a powerful woman?* 'I said it was good,' was his reply.

His anecdote had raised many questions in me. Did ambition and determination constitute power in a woman? If this was something men found daunting, did Seth see himself as a lion tamer? Was he proud to think he was in control of such a woman?

If so, that changed as I grew frenetic in my bid for recognition. 'I wasn't competing with you, Seth,' I responded, more gently. 'I was like a puppy, bringing you a slipper and hoping for a pat on the head. When I didn't get one, I'd look around for a bigger slipper. I got all slippered out.'

I was convinced my hyperactivity had caused my cancer. Had the transformation of his powerful wife into someone needy and, ultimately, very sick and needy, been a turn-off for him?

'I'd do better now,' he said.

His voice was flat. I didn't believe him.

'You're always going to do better, starting tomorrow.' I said. 'Why now?'

'What do you mean?'

'It's been two years,' I reminded him.

'If I didn't do anything before, it's because my pride was hurt.' He shifted in his chair. 'If you could only put all this behind you.'

A voice inside my head was shouting: *Don't listen! This is not him wanting you. He just wants power over you.*

I heard myself say, 'How do I start again, Seth?'

Did he really believe I could do that all on my own, without any effort from him?

'I was thrown away. How would you help me do that?'

He shrugged. 'Dunno.'

He looked like a little boy lost.

That look still had the power to move me. My hard line softened. 'In a way, you're proposing. I suppose you could go down on one knee, like you didn't do the first time.'

As soon as the words left my mouth, I felt like a loser. For any gesture to be worth something, it had to be spontaneous. I was relieved when he threw his hands up in horror.

'I'd never go down on my knees!'

3.

At the end of this meeting, I hadn't forgiven Seth any more than I was reconciled with him.

The Divorce and Separation Recovery Course taught that forgiveness was a process. We could forgive one day and have it all to do over the next, and the next. The important thing was to make a start.

I felt I'd made no start at all. If anything, my feelings were more turbulent than before.

Seth's previous rejection was back in front of my face again, which made me rage. I had also failed in the mission of reconciliation that had been thrust upon me.

This made me want to get away because away from home would be away from him. If I were far away, his failure to call or show up wouldn't be so glaring.

The following weekend, I was glad to get away to attend a

conference of Christian Mission to the Jews (CMJ). Veronica had talked to me about this mission's work. Founded by anti-slavery campaigner, William Wilberforce, CMJ was celebrating its two hundredth anniversary of befriending Jews and supporting their return to their ancestral homeland, Israel.

My kids deplored my getting mixed up in what they saw as yet another cult, (like the Anglican Church), which made me chuckle when I attended the Annual General Meeting, held during the conference. The board was comprised mainly of bosomy English grannies in flowered frocks.

The conference also included a presentation of CMJ's work in Israel. Their guesthouse in Jaffa, near Tel Aviv, was starting an arts discipleship course in September.

I liked the idea of volunteering and receiving training in the arts. I wasn't totally sure what arts discipleship consisted of but I was a picture-maker and a writer and thought I would enjoy the course, as well as have the opportunity to mature in faith.

I was sure Terry would be pleased if I went. Her growing conviction that our ministry would be to the Jews in Israel had been another factor in my opting to attend this conference.

The prospect of being in Israel alone — not on a short visit but for a whole year — terrified me.

I mentioned my dilemma during the conference at the Sunday morning prayer meeting where we prayed for the Nation of Israel. Others prayed for enlightenment for me and for a good decision. I did the same.

Dear God, please direct my feet in the path You would have me follow. If it is Your will that I should join this course, then please facilitate that for me. If You open that door, I will obey. If it is Your will for me to go to Israel, protect me there and allow me to feel at home. Let me not be fearful in my undertakings but trust in You.

I felt a warm glow like sunshine on my face. I was sure God wanted me to go to Israel and take this arts discipleship course.

The literature about it required me to send in an application form and supply two references, one from my pastor and another from a mature Christian. I had only recently joined HTB and didn't have a pastor who knew me well. I would probably have to ask my rabbi...

Ooh, that felt scary. If I did that, my treason might be uncovered. However, I saw that CMJ's guesthouse in Jaffa was called *Beit Immanuel*, (which means House of God Within Us). It was possible that the rabbi might not realise it was Christian.

The rabbi's reference came back fine. My second referee was Veronica. I sent off the application.

4.

I reached in my handbag for my door keys after Tania dropped me at the end of a mother-daughter shopping trip and noticed the bird. It was sitting very still on the wall of the raised flowerbed by my front door.

The bird was a plump wood pigeon, with a pink breast and grey head. The soothing coo of wood pigeons is a common sound in my area. They waddle about my garden and play scared, rising in a half-flutter, whenever a squirrel launches a mock-attack on them.

Whenever I come near, they fly away.

However, this one didn't move as I hoisted myself up to sit on the wall alongside it. 'Well, hello there,' I said. 'How do you do?'

Its beady eye observed me with no trace of fear.

'What a lovely, pink breast you have,' I said, in what I hoped was a reassuring tone. All the while, I was checking it over visually for signs of injury. Seeing none, I assumed it had had a bit of a shock, a mild brush with a vehicle perhaps.

I chatted on for a while, swinging my legs and my door keys at the end of my finger. The wood pigeon was a good listener. However, there were only so many things I could find to say to it.

'Well, this has been nice.' I said, sliding off the wall. 'I'll be going in now. You just sit there as long as you want.'

When I came out to check on the bird, forty minutes later, it was gone.

'Wow!' Terry exclaimed, when I told her about it. 'This is amazing, Bobbie.'

Interesting, yes, I thought. Amazing, no. But she was not done.

'I had a bird encounter, too!'

Now that was something.

'A few days ago, a sparrow flew smack into the plate glass door of the patio. Boom! It dropped onto the deck. At first, I thought it was dead but it was only stunned, so I picked it up and stroked it.'

Talking softly to the bird, she carried it to the safest place she could think of, given that predators teemed in the fields and woods surrounding her home. 'As gently as I could, I put the little sparrow in the cleft between the trunk and a branch of an isolated tree. *You can rest up there until you're good to go*, I told him. I came back to check on him about forty minutes later and he was gone.'

'It's like you and I are living parallel lives,' I said. 'It's like the churches thing, all over again.'

I felt God was drawing my attention to things, turning the mundane into sacred, through this connection to Terry. My Man in the Sky picture would not have grabbed me as strongly as it did, if I hadn't already seen Terry's angel shots. Now this bird experience, which I had seen as anecdotal, was transformed from haphazard into intentional by co-ordinated timing that seemed nothing short of miraculous.

Bero, in Tel Aviv, had told Terry to take care of the fallen birds. Did this encounter signify a further push in that direction for her? And, if these meetings with birds had meanings, what did mine mean?

'That's not all,' she went on. 'My brother Butch also had a bird encounter.'

'Oh, my goodness!' This was astonishing. Three of us at once, Lord?

Though I'd never met this Butch, I recalled that he had been present, so to speak, at King of Kings when Terry took her photos 'for my brother, Butch' who would, 'love this.'

'He was tanning in a park in Fredericton, lying flat out, with his eyes closed,' she began.

'Where's Fredericton?'

'It's where he lives, the capital of New Brunswick,' she said. 'Anyways, the ravens were going crazy over his head, flying this way and that and caw-cawing at one another. He wasn't gonna let them ruin his day. He carried right on lying in the sun, half asleep. Suddenly, something hit his chest with a great thud. He nearly had a heart attack.'

I could picture it: the warm sun, the intense, annoying noise, the fingers curled, waiting for a dollop of bird poop to land on your face, and her brother, with eyes tight shut, determined to ride it out and get some peace.

'Was it a raven?' I pulled a face, horrified and disgusted by the thought of a black bird falling out of the sky onto me.

'That's what he thought. He thought one of them had landed dead on top of him. But, when he opened his eyes, he saw it was his own sandal!' She mimicked a man's voice. 'One of them must have tried to make off with it and found it too heavy. *A person can't tan in the park these days without birds trying to steal your shoes,* he said.'

What could it all mean? 'What did he think about it?'

'He has strong faith but he won't look at it as any kind of a message. He was only relieved not to open his eyes to a pair of coal black wings wrapped around his chest.'

Her imagery made me laugh. At the same time, so many questions were criss-crossing through my brain that I wondered whether these signs and wonders might not be pointers at all but riddles, intended to let me know He had me.

'The ravens fed Elijah,' Terry said. I knew the bible story she was referring to. It was from the First Book of Kings. When that outspoken prophet was in hiding, the ravens brought him *bread and flesh*, twice daily.

'My brother's a nurturer, like those ravens. He earns his living looking after people.'

My take on the ravens dropping a shoe on her brother was more in the nature of a wake-up-and-get-moving type of a call.

'Perhaps he's involved in whatever it is that's happening to us,' I suggested.

'I don't think so.'

I wondered what her reason was for saying that, when our simultaneous bird encounters seemed to indicate the opposite. However, she didn't volunteer an explanation and I didn't ask, at least not directly. 'Is he one of the men pictured on the rug?'

'Definitely not!'

She doesn't want her kid brother included in the game was what crossed my mind. I gave up on that line of enquiry.

'What do you think my bird encounter adds up to, Terry?'

'I think you're going to be flying and loving it. I think you're supposed to go to that place Bero said.'

He had been on my mind lately. I was ashamed of how offhand I'd been with him, when he had shown us only kindness. 'Lake Maggiore?'

'Tell me again where that is,' Terry said.

I had looked it up. 'It's on the Swiss-Italian border.'

'Yep, from there, your next destination for travel will be revealed.'

I really didn't see how I could fit all these trips in, let alone afford them.

5.

'You might have called!' I told Veronica at the door. 'You're an hour late. I might have done something useful with my time, if you'd taken the trouble to let me know.'

She had come to my house for bible study.

'It really is too bad,' I continued, stamping into my living room and leaving her in the hallway to take off her coat. 'You have no consideration.'

I didn't know why I was so angry. It had been a long time since I'd lost my temper like this with anyone. And I really had no reason. Veronica was always late. It had never riled me like this before.

I don't know how I expected her to respond to my outburst but her killer words, delivered in a quite voice, were a shock.

'You are young in faith, Bobbie,' she said, 'just a few months. I'm not sure you're ready for a programme like the one you've applied for.'

She was referring to the arts discipleship course in Israel for which she had supplied a reference.

My reaction to this took me as much by surprise as my flare up. I slumped into an armchair and burst into tears. Veronica knelt down beside me and put her arms around me.

'I can't do it,' I sobbed. 'I can't do what you're asking of me. Seth makes out he wants me but there's no connection between his words and his feet. His words are empty.'

'Then rest,' she said. 'Don't do anything.'

'God doesn't ask something of us that we're incapable of.'

'No, He doesn't.'

Was I hearing correctly: after all her efforts to get me to go back with Seth, she was prepared to leave it?

Her most recent strategy had been to email me extracts from 1 Corinthians 7, where the Apostle Paul writes that women should not separate from their husbands. (Or, if they do, they must remain unmarried.) By staying in the marriage, a believing wife sanctifies an unbelieving husband who is willing to remain with her, and their children are holy.

It looked as if I had made myself wrong with God, which was hard to take. However, when I read the whole chapter, I found that Paul also said that each one should remain in the situation they found themselves in when God called them.

God called me when I was alone.

I dried my eyes and blew my nose. 'I'll have to wait for Him to fill me with forgiveness for Seth, because, clearly, I can't do it on my own.'

Tenderly and earnestly, Veronica began to pray for me. 'Please give Bobbie rest and peace. Lord. '

As she spoke, my anguish slid from my back like a heavy rucksack.

'She cannot resolve this alone. We give Seth up to you, Father God.'

'Amen,' I said. It was a huge relief not to have to deal with this anymore.

Although we were friends again, Veronica's final words to me that evening held a sting. 'I'll pray about whether or not to allow the reference I wrote to stand.'

By now, I wanted very much to be on that arts discipleship course and was sure I would be. If it was within God's plan for me, neither Veronica nor anyone else could prevent it. He would make it happen.

6.

The more I learned about pigeons, the more blessed I felt to have had the opportunity to chat with one.

The wood pigeon was one of four biblical species of dove that, according to all-creatures.org, *is still found today in the forests of Gilead and Carmel*. In the bible, pigeons were used in purification rituals. As a member of the dove family, they also symbolised love and the presence of the Holy Spirit, like the one that flew down to Jesus at His baptism.

It seems strange to caution you not to mistake a bird for a horse... I read in a nineteenth century article, reproduced at www.godweb.org. I was astonished that someone had actually written a piece about the two disparate creatures I was currently concerned with. I couldn't decide which was stranger, my being simultaneously associated with a bird and a horse, or my stumbling upon an article on that very subject.

A horse, it went on, carries us *step by step, by laborious reasoning, into a new state*. Birds, on the other hand, give us a *picture, an idea, of another state*.

On that analysis, the rug, where I was catching prey on horseback, indicated an unfolding role, whereas my chat with a wood pigeon to buck up its spirits was a snapshot of a future me, happy enough in myself to hearten others. I was all for that and looked forward to that.

7.

'The topic for tonight is Moving On,' our group leader at the Divorce and Separation Recovery Course said. 'Can we see ourselves in a new relationship?'

My group comprised of three men and me. I'll call them Matthew, Mark and Luke. A majority of men was unusual, as the course tended to appeal to women. They were good men, who were prepared to admit that they were hurting and needed a helping hand. Getting to know them had helped restore my faith in man-*kind*.

I didn't know what I could say about moving on that wouldn't sound fatuous. I was glad when Peter, our facilitator, turned first to Matthew, who was furthest away from me.

Matthew had his own business in the Home Counties. 'I see that I was too domineering. I'd like to meet a woman young enough to give me another child and start again. I like being a Dad.'

Mark, who always came straight from the office in the same dark blue suit, also said he would like to marry again. He wanted to find a woman with children to bring up. 'I've been a good father,' he told us intently, 'got that much right.'

Luke was still trying to get back with his wife, who was keeping the children from him. It struck me that he was a lot more interested in them than in her.

I was surprised how strongly they all identified themselves through fatherhood. 'All three of you have spoken of renewing that role,' I pointed out, 'rather than of being close to a woman.'

'If I'm not a dad,' Mark told the floor, 'I feel as if I've lost my place in the world.'

'I made an awful hash of being close to a woman,' Matthew chipped in.

I had heard him tell his story and didn't agree. However, I never intended to blurt as I did. 'All that counselling she sent you for, when, clearly, she had no intention of getting back with you, was just to make it look as if it was your fault.'

My cheeks flushed. I thought I'd gone way too far but Peter was nodding. 'We need to get to a place where we're fine again alone, before thinking of dating.'

That sounded right. My little attempts to date had been so awful because I was still bristling about how badly I had been let down. I wasn't ready.

'How do you see moving on, Bobbie?' he asked.

I squirmed a little before making up my mind to speak the truth. 'I can't give out signals,' I said. 'I can't even begin to imagine being able to do that. It's like I'm all tightly packed in a shell, afraid of opening up and becoming vulnerable again.'

Now all four of them were nodding.

'I hate the idea of going through the preliminaries. I don't want to spend a lot of time, only to find it's been a waste of time. What I want is impossible: I want the right person, and I want to know it right away. I want to be straight into a warm, snug place.'

As we left, Peter told me that what I had said to Matthew tonight helped him hugely. Their encouragement as I fumbled to put words to my feelings had helped me, too.

8.

Lampshades hung in smelly tatters. Some creeping disease had shredded every piece of fabric in the holiday flat at Hardelot, a seaside resort in Northern France, where Seth and the kids growing up and I had spent so many long and happy summers.

The flat looked nothing like it used to, which made me sad. When my driver, who was a stranger to me, first pulled up outside the building, a thrill had gone through me. Now I was inside and the family was looking on sadly, as I flapped my hands to shoo away the birds pecking holes in the carpet.

This was some crazy dream.

As the birds rose, Seth pushed them out through a gaping hole in the wall — cracks zigzagged away from it in every direction.

'You should do it up and sell it,' I told him, thinking there would be extra money here that I had not reckoned with, although, judging by the condition of the place, it would not be much.

'I'll do that,' Seth replied.

But all he did was shove wet plaster into the hole, which made the wall look worse. The futility of this makeshift repair was brought home to me by a wind, roaring around my ears. When I turned, the entire wall behind me was gone.

I didn't ask to see this, I thought, as I hurried down the stairs and told my driver to take me away.

I awoke with a start. The yellow light from the streetlamp filtered through my bedroom venetians like the Victorian gaslight setting of a creepy movie. I turned over and tried to sleep, but my dream kept jumping out of the dark shadows at me.

Even so, I noticed that something inside had shifted. When I sought to take out my resentment and examine it, like the woman in the Robert Burns poem who nurses her anger to keep it warm, I discovered a void. To my amazement, all anger had left me. All that remained was a kind of hankering for what had been lost or, rather, what I once thought I had.

I actually found myself smiling at one amusing aspect of the dream. Seth would not know which end of a hammer to pick up. He was no handyman. Suggesting to him to do up the flat was just asking the wrong person. That wasn't his fault. It was just who he was.

Seth was Seth. He could only be himself.

With sudden clarity, I saw that it had been my expectations of him that were all wrong, all along.

I had a choice. I could accept the little he was able to give me or walk away. A person with a choice can't call herself a victim. And, if I wasn't a victim, why should I be angry?

And there it was. Just like that, I was no longer angry with Seth. I did not need to forgive him for there was nothing to forgive.

Accepting what was felt fantastic. I turned over and went back to sleep.

Chapter 7

1.

Far below my sun lounger, boats no bigger than gnats skimmed the water, forming white 'V' shapes in their wake. The church clock in the toy village down by the shore tinkled the quarter hour.

My expectations about this trip to Lake Maggiore were grounded in Terry's assertion that I would receive my next destination for travel here. So far, however, I had received no such thing.

My week's visit was nearly done. In two days, I would exchange the peace God had granted me here for London's traffic and urban sprawl.

A lone man appeared on the lawn by the pool where I was sunbathing. He carefully spread his towel and lay down on top of it. He was rather handsome, if overly tall and thin.

Aha, maybe he was my next destination for travel.

Until now, I had been the only guest staying alone at this simple *pensione*, perched high above the Swiss end of Lake Maggiore. Everyone else here turned out to be couples.

I had observed that, sadly, most had nothing to say to one another. One time, I watched a man and his wife, gazing in opposite directions, like the final photos of Prince Charles and Diana, for two hours.

The man now sharing the lawn with me seemed unable to settle. He fussed with his towel. He turned this way and that. In no time at all, he was on his feet again, calling out to the guy from the house next door, *'Vieni qui! Vieni qui!'* ('Come here.')

I looked around. There was no one else here but me. From his anxious tone, I concluded that the sight of me, lying on a sun lounger, was terrifying him.

The neighbour shouted back. He didn't sound like he was coming.

The man released a flow of words, accompanied by little stamps and the arm waving of an irate toddler. I wondered how anyone could say so much in so little time. But it was all to no avail. The other guy was staying put. Hands on hips, the man fell silent.

With relief, I closed my eyes. The next time I opened them, he was gone.

He had come across to me as a local. (Although this was the Italian part of Switzerland, all the tourists seemed to be German-speaking.) I assumed the owner of the *pensione*, a middle-aged man with drinking buddies in nightly attendance, had tried to set him up with me.

Pensive, I gazed through the gap in the mountains, where the lake flicked a conger eel tail into Italy. All at once, my face creased into a smile: the man's retreat had a lot in common with my own farcical flight from Tel Aviv beach, after a man wanted to chat me up.

Wow, I'd moved on a lot since then — now I was the one scaring men away.

Watching marriage in the middle years here had left me envious of no one. I was content on my own, with my own company.

I didn't see myself with a man right now, not at all. And that was fine.

2.

I had hoped, on my return from Lake Maggiore, to learn whether or not I had been accepted on the arts discipleship course. It was now August and the course started in September. Yet those in charge didn't seem to be in any hurry to reach a decision.

When I prayed about whether I would be going, which I did often, I had no misgivings, despite the possibility that Veronica might have scuppered me by withdrawing her reference.

I was still pretty sure I would be offered a place.

I shared all this with Terry, who sympathized with me.

I had no idea she would take it upon herself to send *Beit Immanuel* a wordy reference, without asking me first. She was trying to help me. However, her reference assumed Veronica had withdrawn hers. It hinted that Veronica didn't know what she was talking about because she didn't understand that we had been given a special mission for Jesus.

I didn't think Terry's intervention had helped my case. It made me look as if I'd chosen the wrong referee in Veronica and was now trying to patch up that blunder. Worse, without a full explanation of what 'a special mission for Jesus' added up to, (something that I, 'an integral part of this', would have been challenged to provide right now), we could be considered delusional.

Days passed. Still I heard nothing.

It got to mid-August. If I was going, I needed to make arrangements about my house. I couldn't just go off and leave it empty.

Frustratingly, I didn't get to speak to anyone on the phone, so I emailed an urgent request for a decision.

The reply came back a no. No reason why was given.

I lay on the couch with my hand covering my eyes. I was hurt and, all at once, exhausted.

I was more upset at having to face the fact that I had been hearing God wrong than I was about not going to Israel or being rejected. If I couldn't rely on what I believed to be God's answer to my prayers, what could I rely upon?

I sent up a prayer about this. 'Why, Father God, did I mishear you and why was I turned down when I thought I would be going?'

I would probably never know for sure whether Veronica had withdrawn her reference or not, since I had no intention of asking her. I might have been turned down because of what Terry wrote or because I put pressure on them for a decision. The reason might have been something else entirely.

I was feeling so sleepy. I could hardly keep my eyes open.

Words that sounded like gibberish popped into my head: *You have to know that they have been scratching the ceiling.*

I didn't know what this might mean so I fired off an email to Terry. Along with the news that I was not now going to Israel, I told her about these strange words.

Bizarrely, they made sense to her. 'The day I got your email, I went down to the basement and heard a heap of scratching in the ceiling,' she told me, when next we spoke. 'It was my cat, Snowball. She'd been missing for several days. She'd had her kittens in amongst the pipes.'

Her interpretation left me none the wiser.

3.

We discussed Bero during that same telephone conversation.

'I wrote him an email several days ago,' Terry told me. 'I haven't had a reply.'

'I emailed him, too,' I replied.

'You did?'

My conscience was pricking me before leaving for Lake Maggiore. I emailed Bero at the Tel Aviv hotel where he worked. 'I thanked him for his suggestion of Lake Maggiore as a destination and apologised for being frosty when I was in Israel. He replied that he was glad to have been of some help.'

It was no big deal. I probably wouldn't have mentioned the

exchange to Terry, if she hadn't brought Bero up.

After a pause, she said, 'Maybe I won't hear back. Maybe his work is done.'

'That was what I was thinking,' I said.

As soon as Terry said she'd had no reply to her email, I had the strongest impression she wouldn't. That Bero had done what he had to do, as far as we were concerned, and moved on.

4.

'I was all psyched up for Israel,' I told my new friends, Paul and Cindy, who had come to my house for supper. 'I even dreamt I was going. Did I hear God all wrong?'

This mature Christian couple in their forties had attended the CMJ Conference two months before. Paul was involved in preparing CMJ's newsletter.

Veronica, who had made the original introductions during her home church's tent outreach week, was also here.

Paul blinked. 'Didn't you say you found the idea of being in Israel alone quite frightening?'

'Yes, I did.' He had a good memory. It was something I'd mentioned driving home from the conference in their car.

We were sitting at the table in my pale blue dining room. It was a beautiful summer's evening. Scents of rose and honeysuckle were drifting in through the open patio door.

'Perhaps God wanted to see if you'd go through with it,' Cindy suggested. She was very proper, popping one pea at a time onto the end of her fork and into her mouth.

Paul beamed at his wife. 'Like Abraham, when he was told to sacrifice his son, Isaac?'

'Precisely,' she said. 'God was testing his commitment and obedience. He didn't actually mean him to go the whole hog.'

'You're saying that, knowing I had misgivings about being there alone, God wanted to see if I was sufficiently obedient to go anyway?' I asked.

'And, like Abraham, you were let off the hook at the last minute,' Paul said.

I glanced at Veronica, sitting beside me. She was uncharacteristically quiet this evening. Knowing how upfront she always was, I was pretty sure she would have told me, if she had decided to withdraw the reference she wrote for me. I concluded, from her silence, that she had not.

'I suppose I've been shown what I'm not required to do,' I conceded. 'But how am I to discern what God does want?'

Cindy dabbed delicately at her lips with her napkin. 'Prayer and trying doors. The right ones will open.'

I gathered up the knives and forks and dinner plates. I brewed coffee in the kitchen and brought bowls of fresh fruit salad.

It grew dark as we talked about this and that, the unaccustomed stillness I had enjoyed at Lake Maggiore, Paul's love of Christian music…

Eventually, I brought the conversation full circle, back to my not hearing God right. I guess it still bothered me.

'Of course, it could all be a question of timing,' Paul threw in.

His words sounded like nothing more than a sweetener.

'A no now could be a yes later,' Cindy said.

Paul blinked in my direction. 'You may be meant to go to Israel, just not right away.'

'Sometimes, God's will seems to be coming to me through a lot of static,' I admitted with a sigh.

Insects had begun crowding in to commit *hari kiri* by throwing themselves against the overhead light. Little black corpses were dropping into our empty coffee cups. I got up to slide the patio door shut.

As I did so, a realisation came to me. If I was not yet able to discern the things of the Kingdom that I needed to know without the support and training I was receiving through HTB and the advice of mature Christians like Paul and Cindy, I was probably not yet ready to go on a course to learn how to disciple others.

Veronica had been right in her assertion that I was too young in faith for that course.

Paul suggested we end with a prayer.

'That would be lovely,' I said.

He bowed his head. 'Dear God, thank you for the good food and lively conversation we have enjoyed at this table tonight and thank you, too, for the fellowship we have shared. Bless Bobbie, as she remains in her house…'

I breathed in the still peace that had descended on the room.

'…and bless us as we take the road tonight. Grant her peace and contentment in her home, continue to fill it with warmth and laughter. I ask, Lord, that You would bless this house. May Bobbie always be aware of Your Loving Presence here and may she clearly hear everything You wish to tell her. Thank you, Lord. Amen.'

'Amen,' I said, bursting with excitement.

It had happened, just as Terry had said. Someone had appeared to bless my house.

I was amazed and overjoyed.

I'd just completed a two-week intensive course in Hebrew. The spontaneous blessing of my house had been the last outstanding element of her night dictation to me in Tel Aviv. I hadn't thought it could happen but it had.

5.

I liked that many couples of all ages attended the services at Holy Trinity Brompton, (HTB). They praised God and sat close to hear the sermon together.

I wanted some of that. It would be good to be deep in faith with a husband, I thought.

On the train home from worship at HTB this particular August Sunday, I stared out of the dust-smeared window as the Thames, bathed in silver rays of evening sunlight, and the disintegrating shell of Battersea Power Station rattled past. The sermon tonight had encouraged us to take time out to be with God. It was something we could do at home or anywhere, like sitting on a train.

As the bronze statues of waiting passengers on the platform at Brixton slipped by, a message came into my head: *I will send someone for you.* No heavenly music, no tingles down my spine. The words came like a voice, speaking plainly to me. I had the immediate conviction that it spoke truth.

To receive a word, any word, from God is beautiful. I might have been strolling alongside turquoise waters, rather than rocked this way and that by a dingy suburban train, such was the peace that filled me. I had trouble suppressing a smile. The leggy teenager, lolling opposite, checked himself as he half smiled back.

I had wondered at Chanelle's prayer: 'Dear Lord, accept this woman as your obedient bride and, when the time is right, please provide her with a new earthly husband.'

I had been unable then to imagine being with a man. But God took me as I came to Him, angry and broken, and cradled me in His strong arms, until I was comforted.

'You will dance again,' Chanelle had said.

Now God seemed to be saying this, too.

As the train carriage criss-crossed tracks and passengers chatted on mobile phones, the voice in my head continued:

The man I have for you is in the world, doing his best, through his work, to make a mitzvah, (do good). He's a good man, who's thoughtful and calm. He'll love to learn. He'll love looking at stuff with you and sharing ideas. He'll be quietly handy, a home-loving homemaker.

And he was already out there, hoping to meet me.

'Could he please be kind,' I requested, 'as well as one of Yours?'

I needed kind.

The sunshine on my face feeling that followed confirmed that he would be.

Rounding a long bend, to the squeal of brakes, we lurched forward and back in our seats. My stop was next.

'Sorry,' I told the teenager as I scrambled to my feet and almost fell on top of him.

This time, he smiled for real.

Though it was a hot, sticky evening, I fairly skipped up the station steps to Bromley High Street. I had looked to God to glue my broken dreams together for me. Now I saw that He was giving me new dreams.

'Just trust and wait until His sign shows you your path,' Chanelle had said.

One day, when the time was right, I would meet the man God had for me. How far ahead that lay didn't seem to matter. I did not need to know when or where. By putting myself where I belonged, he would appear. It would happen in God's good time and His timing is always perfect.

I had almost reached my front door before I thought to add an extra request. 'Please, Lord, if at all possible, could he also be fanciable?'

It would be perfect if the outside looked as good as the inside.

6.

I wanted to see Terry's home and meet her husband and little boy. Above all, I wanted very much to see the rug. Since I was no longer tied up with an extended trip to Israel, I could.

I decided go to Canada. The flights would be the longest I'd taken since before my lung clots.

When I invited myself to stay for twelve days, starting next week, Terry was gratifyingly excited. 'Wow, that's fantastic! There's so much to catch up on, Bobbie.'

Her words gave me a warm feeling inside.

She came up with yet another prophecy for me. 'I just got the strongest feeling that God wants to show you something on your way here.'

'That's great,' I said, accepting that a communication from God as I travelled was possible, even likely. I believed He had called me. I believed He loved me. In just a few months, scepticism and mistrust had given way to acceptance that God could and would tap me on the shoulder frequently and by any means. I treasured that connection.

Chapter 8

1.

On 31st August, 2007, I flew to Halifax, Nova Scotia. From there, I boarded what would turn out to be a very slow train, so slow that I could probably have beaten it, walking alongside. My destination was Moncton, New Brunswick.

I found my seat and sat, making up a little story in my head, as I waited for it to pull out of Halifax.

My story was about a bird's egg that fell into a lake. The baby bird could see its surroundings through the shell. When it hatched, it whooshed to the surface and up, into the air. There was no real story to it. It was more of a situation. What I liked was that the bird had actually enjoyed being in an alien environment. It missed the fishes and wafting seaweed.

The train conductor was in front of me, imposing in dark uniform and cap. He checked my ticket and said, 'Would you like to be the Able-Bodied Saviour?'

His accent was Eastern European.

To be nominated Able-Bodied Saviour sounded pretty wonderful. Without any idea what was involved, I said, 'Yes.'

He led me to the train doors at the end of the compartment and went through the emergency evacuation procedure.

So this was what he meant. I nodded and grinned as he showed me everything.

When he was done, he led me back to my seat. 'So now it's official,' he said. 'You are the Able-bodied Saviour.'

He took out a pen and wrote on a yellow post-it note that he stuck on the luggage rack, above my head. As soon as he walked away, I jumped up to read it. Sure enough, it said: *Able-bodied Saviour.*

I was definitely that person: I had a yellow post-it note to prove it.

I had fretted about the long flight this journey required and did all the deep vein thrombosis prep — aspirin, surgical stockings, drank loads of water during the flight and kept moving. Everything had gone without a hitch. I felt great.

Being nominated Able-Bodied Saviour seemed to be a confirmation from God that I had no cause to worry about travelling.

Terry had told me something special would happen on my journey to her place. This was pretty special. I felt God was already blessing this visit.

2.

Terry, Don and nine-year old Lonnie met me at Moncton Station. Don's black beard was streaked with grey. He had blue eyes and looked as strong as a lumberjack. Lonnie was small for his age and slight.

Terry and I hugged and laughed, joyful to be reunited.

During supper in a diner, Don jawed endlessly about himself. Lonnie said very little. What he did say was in an accent I found hard to understand.

They lived an hour's drive into the countryside. We passed villages, wooden churches and scrubby farms along the way.

I was eager to see the rug.

As soon as we reached the house, a large and elegant log cabin at the end of a long drive, Terry directed me upstairs to where it hung on the wall in a dark area, to protect it from fading.

It was exquisite. And the accuracy of our likenesses was beyond comprehending. I gazed and gazed.

To stand before the real thing was an otherworldly experience, like passing through the wardrobe into a lost kingdom of sultans, where I hurtled towards Terry on a red Arabian, with the wind on my face and the nutty smell of horse sweat in my nostrils. Everything around me — creatures, branches, plants — was on the move.

Now I stood before the real thing, I could see what I couldn't see in photos. The lovely soft gleam under lamplight of the buttery gold background, for instance. But I could also see a negative: it had not been looked after very well and must have been stored folded, rather than rolled. A ridge ran down the middle where the silk threads had worn.

I ran my hand across the pile. It had the smooth texture of freshly-shampooed hair.

I loved this rug.

Its execution was exuberant and joyful, even though some of the elements of the story were really rather gruesome, like the shooting of an ibex with a bow and arrow and preparing to skin a deer. It was good that the two murderous men were facing away from the action, about to exit the scene.

Terry came and stood beside me. Shoulder to shoulder, we gazed at the rug.

'There I am,' I said to her, in a hushed tone of wonder.

'There you are.'

'And there you are, galloping gleefully in my direction.'

She was clearly depicted as the bearer of good news.

'I'm heralding the Christian faith to the Jews,' she said.

As far as I knew, I was the only Jew she had ever heralded to.

3.

Later that evening, the two of us decided to go for a walk. Given that signs and wonders happened when we were together, I should not have been surprised at the way this turned out.

We could choose between their hundred acres of dense woodland out back, where we might run into bear, or the track to the road, where we might run into what Terry called 'rednecks.'

We chose the latter. It felt good to be out in the countryside. We strolled past farms. The fields were filled with wild flowers, under the slanting sun. We didn't meet any joyriders. Ours was an encounter of a different kind.

'Maybe we'll see deer,' Terry said. 'I see them everywhere when I go out with my family or driving.'

I pointed out some red-brown shapes in the long grass at the back of a broad field, rimmed by trees. 'There are some.'

'Oh, my goodness!' She headed straight off in their direction, across the pasture that bordered the road. 'Come on.'

There was no signed footpath like in England here. We had to be trespassing. I feared someone might appear toting a rifle. 'Won't the farmer mind?'

'Oh, no, he's our neighbour.'

The deer lifted their heads as we reached the edge of their field. There were four of them.

'Two does and two babies,' I said.

Terry grinned at me. 'When I told the people in Jerusalem I'd never seen so many deer in my life as this year, they said, *We know. More have been added, for protection.*'

She saw herself as being under attack from Satan's fallen angels. I didn't know what to make of that idea, so I said nothing.

One of the deer grunted throatily, a bull-like belch. We stopped.

'It's calling to us,' Terry said.

'Yes.'

They began to run towards us, which seemed very strange.

'They're running towards us, Terry!'

'Yes!' She sounded thrilled.

They had to be does, since they had no horns and they had babies. But I could not think of a single reason why does with babies to protect would run towards us. Maybe I was wrong and they were stags. I knew stags sometimes attacked humans during the rutting season, which was now.

'They are does, aren't they?'

'They're does,' she confirmed.

They came to a halt a hundred or so yards from us and stared with giraffe necks. We stared back.

'I think.'

'You *think*?' In my mind, this was hardly the time to be making assertions you were unsure of. The deer had already shown themselves to be unpredictable.

'Stay still, Bobbie.'

'I'm not going anywhere.' I kept my eyes on the deer.

The one that spoke to us before grunted again, a short bark, deep and hollow. Receiving no answer from us, it repeated the sound and, a few seconds later, did it a third time. The deer seemed to be losing patience with us.

'Should we answer?' It seemed rude not to.

'Do you speak deer?' Terry asked.

'Ha, ha.'

'I think they want to be friends.'

'Oh-oh, they're running towards us again!'

It seemed as if they might really attack us.

They were sixty or seventy yards from us and closing when Terry flicked at the growing swarm of midges around our heads. These annoying bugs were intent on exploring our every orifice.

The deer peeled off in the direction of the sweep of her hand. They wheeled right around the field, springing through the long grass at the back, before disappearing into the trees.

I attempted a grunt.

Terry threw up her arms. 'Why didn't you say that before?'

4.

Terry made a good story of our deer encounter when she dropped me off at her friend Corinne's weekend cabin, a few days later. I had no idea what to make of what happened.

To Terry, that didn't seem to matter. As she told it, 'The deer came real close to us.'

Next time around, she'd probably say we could see their flaring nostrils.

Her exaggeration didn't detract from the fact that it was an extraordinary story.

Terry left soon after telling it. She had errands to run. I would be spending the day here with Corinne, a neat, dark-haired, petite Acadian French woman of about fifty.

The cabin sat on five acres of neat lawn in an idyllic location, above a broad river, deep in the New Brunswick countryside.

But the weather that day was terrible. And, as driving rain beat against the chilly cabin's windows, misery poured out of Corinne, whose husband had been tragically killed right here in a quad bike accident, two years before. She was lonely, she was hard-up. Above all, she was worn out trying to keep everything in good order. And no wonder. She had a further three acres of garden at home to tend, as well as the lawn that surrounded her camper trailer, near the coast.

'I spend all my time going from one to the other and mowing the grass.'

Was it my imagination or had the smell of new-mown grass seeped into her skin? I thought I detected a faint whiff of it as she sat beside me.

'Why do that?'

She was so little. How could she cope with such a huge chore?

'To honour my husband.'

It seemed to me Corinne was not so much honouring her dead husband as denying he'd gone by keeping things exactly as they were when he was alive. She could come to any one of their homes and kid herself he might still walk through the door.

'Sell one,' I suggested. 'Sell everything and get a condo.'

She looked around her at the plank walls and rustic furniture. 'That would be hard. So many memories. And people would say I was forgetting him. Or that I was squandering his money.'

'People', I discovered, were a large clan of family and in-laws who made it their business to 'watch over her', as she put it.

'But it's your money now.'

She shook her head.

This visit was a reminder how people who seem fine on the surface, may not be on the inside. Corinne, like her homes, looked neat and tidy and together, yet, behind the sociable smile, she was on a mudslide.

5.

A few days later, Terry and I set out for Fredericton, New Brunswick's capital, to visit her brother, Butch.

Our vehicle broke down on the Salmon River Road. My initial feeling was relief that this hadn't happened twenty minutes before, when we were going up and down tracks, past camps and cottages, looking for bears, after I'd mentioned that I'd love to see one.

The pick-up Terry was driving was not her regular vehicle but part of the commercial fleet Don ran for his log home building business. Her car was in the garage for repairs, having become unreliable. When the pick-up puttered to a halt and refused to restart, we realised it, too, was unreliable.

Terry couldn't get a signal on her cell phone.

'Don't worry, Bobbie.' She reached for her purse on the back seat.

Until that moment, I hadn't been. I looked around and realised there were only trees and a ribbon of deserted road and I began to worry. I worried about being found by wild animals or wild men. I also worried about not being found at all.

'I know some people who live a few hundred yards back.'

Phew, that was a relief.

However, as we rounded the corner on foot, the burned-out shell of a building came into view.

Terry was not as horrified to see this as I was. She knew all about it and explained that this had been a popular destination for the snowmobiling fraternity, including Don and herself, until a catastrophic kitchen fire earlier that year had wiped out both the café and the owners' home, over top.

'They have guest cottages out back,' she said. 'They've moved into one of those.'

But there was no sign of a car and no answer when we knocked at one of the cottage doors.

'There's a public call box in the car park at the front,' I said.

We returned to the roadside. Terry put in a quarter and gave her number. The operator wanted $3.80 for a one-minute call to Ron, who was home for a few days. Amazingly, I had that amount in quarters and dimes. I passed her the coins and, one by one, she fed them into the slot.

When we were connected, she quickly told Don that we had

broken down near Tia and Tony's café and that her cell phone had no signal.

'What do you want me to do?' I heard Don ask.

'Come and get us, of course!'

The line went dead. Our minute was up.

'*What do you want me to do?*' she mimicked.

At my suggestion, we sat on a low wall, in case Don called back.

After a couple of minutes, she got to her feet. 'There's no point sitting here. I've just remembered public phones in New Brunswick don't take incoming calls.'

She was wrong. The phone rang as we started walking away. Don wanted the full lowdown on what was wrong with the pick-up so he could bring the right parts.

He said he would come as soon as he could.

I had no idea when that might be. The roads here in New Brunswick were long. It would be a while. I followed her out back again with heavy step, frustrated over the chunk of our day we were about to 'lose'.

She looked at me and shrugged. 'It is what it is.'

I wished I could be more easy-going, like she was. Her sunny acceptance made things look brighter.

It helped that we were trapped in a place of outstanding beauty. The wooden outdoor chairs where we sat, with the grass tickling our toes, were on a broad carpet of lawn, perched above a slow-moving river as blue as lapis lazuli. Our little oasis was hemmed in by thick, emerald forest on every side.

All at once, my frustration left me. I had simply reminded myself that God was in control. The calm that came in was balm.

After barely an hour, relaxing in this tranquil spot, a car drew up.

6.

Terry's friends, Tia and Tony, were a lively couple in their late fifties. Unfazed by our unscheduled visit to the small cabin where they were currently living, they worked as a team to make us welcome, brewing coffee and preparing food for us. Small wonder their cafe had been popular.

The four of us sat down to a delicious lunch, to which Terry brought a dramatic retelling of our deer story.

She then asked about incoming calls to payphones.

'Public phones in New Brunswick don't take incoming calls,' Tony said.

'Yours does.' She explained how Don called us back.

'Well, it don't do that,' he asserted.

'That's what I thought,' Terry said. 'But it did. Bobbie was with me.'

'It rang. It was Don,' I confirmed.

The New Brunswick payphone that rang when it wasn't supposed to was looking like the latest way God had chosen to make His Presence felt to Terry and me.

The conversation moved to discussing the effects of the fire on Tia and Tony's life.

Tia missed the life she had before. 'I threw my heart and soul into this place. And we had such times here.'

To my surprise, since they seemed such a solid couple, Tony countered, 'It was hard work.'

'I liked the work.'

The local wildlife had also enchanted Tia. She told us of bears that would wander past their door and raccoons that begged for food on the patio. She described the antics of a pet chipmunk...

It sounded wonderful.

'I'll be leaving all kinds of memories behind,' she said.

They had a buyer for the property, Tony explained. He wanted the burned-out building demolished.

Tia looked downcast. 'It's the end of an era.'

'But she's sick,' Tony said. 'She can't do it no more.'

I was shocked to learn that Tia had lupus and was about to begin a course of chemotherapy. It seemed a harsh blow to lose her health on top of their livelihood and the environment she cherished.

Fire or no fire, I could see she would have had no other choice than to give up the café, anyway.

'Do you know yet what you'll do?' I asked.

'Whatever is God's will is okay with me,' Tia said.

I wasn't convinced she meant that.

Tony explained their ideas. 'We wanna buy some land over by Grand Lake and build some condos to sell to the summer people, so we can manage them for them, when they're not around.'

'That sounds like a good plan,' I said.

'I can't get no enthusiasm for it, though, dear,' she said. 'Man, I'll sure miss it here.'

'Not me,' Tony said. 'I can't wait.'

I was sad this likeable pair weren't in accord.

At this point, Don finally arrived. Tia and Tony both got to their feet to brew fresh coffee. They fed us a fine supper. Then Don and Tony went and fixed the pick-up.

The day was ending when we said our goodbyes.

Tony had a parting warning for us, about a moose he'd seen earlier on the Salmon River Road. 'The biggest moose ever, back there. He was a giant. You'd best take care, now, if you're headed that way.'

I felt a long way from London. Terry reassured me that we were headed in the opposite direction from the moose.

She then suggested prayer before leaving. We prayed for Tia and Tony's restoration. Silently, I also prayed for their restitution as a couple. Tony needed to understand the depth of Tia's attachment to this place. Tia needed to accept that Tony was worn out.

'While you were praying, I got a picture of lakes and hills covered in pine trees,' Tia said, looking happy tearful. 'New Brunswick, bathed in sunshine. It felt real good.'

7.

There had been good weather days here. One blistering day, I even swam in a rock pool of a fast-flowing river. Today wasn't one of those days, however. I was snuggling into the couch with a throw tugged up to my neck as rain ran down the den windows like tears.

Terry peered out at the meadow. 'They have a saying here: *If you don't like the weather, wait five minutes.* But this looks like it's set in for the day. We'll read and study and go see my brother another day.'

I wasn't sorry we were aborting this second attempt at reaching Fredericton. It would have been a long drive. Everywhere was.

'It'll be cosy, just you, me and him,' I said, pointing at the black bearskin that leered up at us from the floor.

We had the house to ourselves. Lonnie was back at school during the day. Don was gone away again, building a log cabin for a client in St. John, a hundred and fifty miles away.

Terry would have been spending a lot of time on her own, if I weren't here. I wouldn't have liked that much but she seemed okay with it. Loneliness wasn't something she talked about. But, then, Terry never talked about things she found challenging.

We began with prayer. She bowed her head and asked for enlightenment for us.

'I had a vision last night concerning you,' she said, when we had finished. Every morning, she had something new to share with me. I was still sceptical of her prophecies, even though pretty much everything she had told me since King of Kings had turned out to be spot on. 'I saw the place where you were living.'

'I've prayed about where God wants me,' I said. 'The answer I get is more about a state of mind: *I want you happy. It will be where you want it.*'

'That's exactly right, Bobbie!' She flung her arms wide. 'You've talked about loving the countryside. I saw slopes of sage green, going down to water that shimmered in the sun.'

'That sounds lovely.'

I wasn't convinced I could live in the countryside, however. From what I'd seen here, the manual work would be too hard, without a man to help me.

'It was lovely,' she said. 'And, off to the left were trees, olive trees.'

'Ah, you're thinking Israel?' I was a little weary of being prodded in that direction.

'The north of the country, perhaps. Around Galilee it was so green.'

'I just tried to go to Israel, Terry, and was turned down. If it had been right, that door would have opened for me.'

8.

Terry was very taken with some prophecy she had received from three men and a woman at the Soulfest Christian Music Festival in New Hampshire, USA, a month previously.

'I only popped my head into their tent to say "hi" on my way to the concert,' she said. 'They were sitting on hard-backed chairs in a circle. They said, *Come on in*, so I did. Boy, it was some hot in there.'

She played me the tape, several times.

'God is shifting and rearranging things in your life,' an American-accented male began.

'If they only knew!' she interjected, pointing upstairs, in the direction of the rug and winking at me.

We both laughed.

The second male voice was younger and had a southern drawl. 'I feel that something's just around the corner. And it's HUGE!'

'Hear that, Bobbie?' Terry said. 'HUGE was the word the rabbi in Jerusalem used.'

'I know.'

Terry clicked the cassette player's pause button. 'This is where the older man, the one who just talked about shifting and rearranging, opened his eyes and leaned forward to look at my ring finger. His eyebrows shot up when he saw my wedding ring.'

She clicked it back on again.

'I was feeling like you're not married, but you are?' he said.

'Yes, I am,' I heard Terry say on the tape.

'But your husband is not in the same place as you spiritually?'

'No, he's not.'

Don was a Jehovah's Witness.

All I could hear now was what sounded like the whirring of a fan, backed by the distant whine of electric guitars.

'This is where they all closed their eyes again and prayed,' she told me.

Eventually, I heard the girl's voice. 'Your husband doesn't get what is happening.'

'I'm hearing that you should look past him to the Lord as your husband, for more purity,' the older man said. 'Purity is the key, purity in heart, word and deed.'

'Your husband's confusion should not deter you,' the girl said.

All this sounded like the reverse of the prayer for a new husband for me that Chanelle had prayed in Jerusalem.

'Thank you, Jesus,' I heard Terry say on the tape.

'Let your actions speak for you,' the older man advised. 'Lessen your words.'

Terry blinked at me. 'I promised myself to stop yelling. Yelling does no good at all.'

She'd forgotten about that when we returned from looking at a piece of her land Don had allowed to get overgrown.

'Y'all are a woman who knows the times and the seasons,' the southerner said.

The fourth one spoke for the first time. 'I'm getting the word "pursue", pursue and not give up.'

'A picture of the rug came into my head at that moment,' Terry told me. 'I saw myself on that running horse with my arms spread wide.'

'I feel like I want to give thanks for Terry!' the southerner exclaimed.

'That's it,' she said and clicked the machine off. 'It was the strangest thing, Bobbie. He got up and hugged me close, like I was going on a long journey and he was sorry to see me go... What do you think?'

As so often happened around things concerning Terry, I didn't know what to think. She seemed inspired by what they had said but their message didn't seem to add up to anything concrete, other than it was as if she weren't married.

As to that, there'd been a few slammed doors since my arrival, as well as the row over the neglected land. She'd sold off her horses a while back. It wouldn't surprise me if that was where she was heading.

'You two aren't getting on, are you?' I said tentatively.

Her dark brown eyes narrowed. 'See that deck out there?' She pointed at a half-finished extension to the rain-splashed patio. 'He started that last May. But it's just been left. I've asked and asked him to finish it but he takes no notice. It'll stay like that now for years.'

As far as I could see, he was working hard, doing his best to earn a living in the months the weather allowed him to. I didn't think her complaints were justified.

'He finishes nothing.' Exasperated, she flopped in her chair like a raggedy doll.

I was no fan of Don's. I found him a dull man who thought himself fascinating. His eyes lingered overlong on the ladies, including myself. Even so, what I said next was unforgivable. 'I think you expect too much. He's a draught horse. You want a thoroughbred and he can't be that.'

I clamped my hand across my big mouth. My cheeks turned to flames. 'That was terrible. I should never have said that.'

'It's okay, Bobbie. You're right.' She seemed completely unperturbed by my rash words.

'I'm so sorry, Terry.' However I writhed, I could not unsay what I had said.

'It's okay. *Really*.' She looked as if it really was. 'I'll stay and make the best of it. I won't be leaving him.'

9.

The following Sunday, Terry held a friends' get-together in honour of my visit. Corinne came, along with others I'd not previously met: Lilly, Heidi and Sarah.

Sarah was a beautiful, young woman with long black hair. She looked like a young Nelly Furtado, the Canadian singer. She spoke to me of her dream to create a camp for kids. 'But I don't know where to begin.'

'Maybe we could pray for the right people to be put in front of you,' I said.

She thought that was a good idea. But her smile soon turned to a frown again. 'I'm not a very together person. I've been told I've built a sandcastle for my home.'

Her husband, though a Christian, had trouble keeping away from the porn sites. Earlier, when we prayed in a circle, her hand in mine made me think of waves and wind, someone all at sea.

'I suppose I should put a fence around it,' she said.

I favoured solid construction over defence. 'You could try rebuilding it with brick or wood.'

My words to Sarah weren't clever or even original, but she looked so encouraged, I felt I had been given the right ones.

'I'll be praying for God's help,' Sarah told me.

'Pray for guidance,' I said and squeezed her hand.

At that moment, Terry came into the living room with a plate of bread and olives. She put it on the table and joined us on the sofa. 'So, who's going next?'

We had been taking turns to share our stories.

'Heidi?' she suggested.

Heidi was a little older than Sarah, in her thirties. Her hair was long, with blond highlights and she had kind eyes. They looked as if they wanted to smile but it was a struggle.

'Okay,' she said and told us that she had recently returned from working Out West in Alberta, where so many Canadians go in search of the big money heavy industry pays there. As she began to speak of the unhappiness within her marriage and the guilt that was weighing her down, she broke down in tears.

'Come with me' Terry said, and led her into another room.

Whatever ministering to broken birds Terry did there had a positive effect. When they returned, Heidi had her smile back.

We all tucked into the yummy spread of roast chicken, pasta and salad Terry had prepared and, afterwards, descended to the basement to croon over kittens. These were the very kittens that had been scratching at the ceiling of Terry's basement.

I reached into the curled up balls of fur out for the white one I'd fallen in love. 'I still don't get what that word I had was all about.'

Terry grinned 'You will. You were meant to come and meet them.' She turned to the others. 'Anybody who wants can have one.'

I held little Snowy, as I had named him, tightly to me. I would have loved to take him home.

'Love kittens, *hate* kitty litter,' Lilly, a bible bookshop employee, said. She and Terry were good friends. They had gone to Soulfest, a US Christian music festival, together that August.

Lilly, who was chubby and mumsy, with black curly hair and blue eyes, had already shared her story. She told us how proud she was that, two years earlier, she had waited until her wedding night to sleep with her second husband. He was not initially happy about this, she said, even though he was a staunch Christian, like she was. He had gone along with it under protest.

Coming, as I did, from liberal, secular England, I didn't know whether I was initially more surprised by the position she had taken or the pride she obviously took in having taken it. A previously-married woman holding out reflected an aspect of Christianity that had not, so far, come up at HTB, either in the worship or on the Divorce and Separation Recovery Course.

I could not imagine going to the altar without first having the comfort of knowing the disfigurement cancer had left me with would not be an issue in the marriage bed. Wondering up to the wire whether a fiancé might show me some of the revulsion I'd sensed in Seth would be more than I could endure, I thought.

An option, I supposed, as my mind ran on, would be to allow pre-marital petting to address the problem. This conjured memories of awkward teenage fumbling in the dark that made me squirm. If that train were set in motion at my age, I was sure that it would be all but impossible to stop it.

Lilly had a right to be proud of her willpower, I decided. There was something pure and beautiful in what she had pulled off.

Cuddling a kitten, Lilly, who also taught Sunday School, asked me about the Jewish Festival of *Sukkot*, or Tabernacles, that was just around the corner. 'I'd like to explain it to my pupils.'

I told her about decorating the *sukkah*, a kind of lean-to, with leaves and fruit and vegetables. 'It smells wonderful. Many Jews build their shelter in their yard or on their balcony and eat and sleep in it.'

She was pleased with this information. I was pleased with her interest in Jewish festivals. When I taught children at Jewish Religion School, the curriculum didn't reference any other faith.

'The difference, I guess, is Jesus was Jewish,' she said. Lilly was trying to deepen the children's understanding of Him by exploring what He celebrated.

Little Lonnie held up a charcoal kitten. 'I'd like to keep dis one,'

'Sorry, honey,' Terry said. 'They're all looking for homes. Who wants one?'

'Kitty litter!' Lilly cried. 'I have to keep reminding myself or I'll be tempted.'

10.

When we went back upstairs, everyone clamoured for my story. I began by telling them how I'd said *hineini*, 'here I am,' because I wanted God to give me purpose in my life. They laughed when I said Terry had called me a 'stinker' because I was going to Israel and she loved Israel. The next thing I knew, she had arranged to come with me.

I described our search for spirituality all over the Land and how, paradoxically, we found it in hectic Jerusalem, in the vibrant King of Kings congregation, and in the Prayer Tower, afterwards.

I tried to convey how it felt to experience the Holy Spirit and spoke of the signs and wonders we had seen, beginning with the strange pictures in Terry's camera that looked like angels.

I conceded that these might have been nothing at all, a glitch in her camera, except for their timing — right as I found myself doing something unprecedented, worshiping at a Jerusalem church — and the fact that they hadn't appeared in isolation — I later discovered my Man in the Sky photo, taken the day before her pictures.

More importantly, these had led Terry, who had pursued their meaning, to a rug, woven before we were born, on which the two of us figured, pursuing deer and rabbits.

I recounted how I had returned home from Israel, still struggling and kicking, so to speak, and arguing that Jesus was no greater than Gandhi. In the end, however, I no longer disputed that He was the Messiah and I welcomed Him into my heart.

This generated a sigh of pleasure, followed by a round of applause.

I spoke of my new relationship of trust with God as my Father and how it had made me a calmer, pleasanter, more accepting person who could forgive my ex and move on.

Beginning at King of Kings, I had signed up for a mission, the detail of which was still to be revealed to me but which I knew would bring me fulfilment. I trusted God to show me my direction in His good time.

'It was the rug that brought me here,' I ended. 'The rug will point the way.'

'It's upstairs,' Terry threw in.

Lilly gaped. 'It is?'

'Would you like to see it?'

Instantly, they were all on their feet, converging on the staircase. There were exclamations of wonder all round when they stood before the rug that hung on the wall opposite my bedroom door.

Heidi looked from us to the rug and back again. 'It's you guys, for sure, both of you!'

The others agreed.

'Don says it's just an old rug,' Terry said. 'He says I'm delusional, that that's not even me on it.'

There had been a cold front between them during the days before Don left for St. John.

'But it is clear,' Corinne said. 'It *is* you!'

'What's the story?' Lilly asked.

'I don't know,' I said. During all the time I had stood staring at it here, nothing new about its meaning had come to me.

'It was made in 1952 by the Mizrahi tribe,' Terry said.

'*Mizrahi* is Hebrew for east. It's a generic term for Jews from the Middle East,' I said. 'My ex was a Mizrahi Jew, from Egypt.'

'The people who made this rug live in Israel now,' she said.

'I guess life wouldn't be too comfortable for a Jew in Iran today,' I said.

I put one arm around Terry on my right and Sarah, who happened to be the person on my left. Though I hardly knew these women, I felt a deep connection to them. 'I'm so glad the rug brought me here.'

'We're glad, too,' Sarah said and the others agreed.

Night had fallen. We went downstairs to share a final prayer, for blessing on our lives and safety on our journeys.

'Please keep the moose off the road,' Lilly prayed, which was not something you'd hear in England.

As their cars pulled away, down the long, winding track that led to the road, it came to me that this was not any kind of a holiday. I was here to learn how to hearten fallen birds.

11.

I came from what had become my daily kitten-cuddle fix to sit on the back deck of Terry's huge log home. I looked out over the meadow where, yesterday, I had gathered armfuls of wild flowers for the girls' get-together.

At the place where the Pony Express rider once used to ford the river at the back of the meadow were the ruins of an old homestead. Out front of their property, in addition to Don's sawmill and the barn, was the hundred-year old house where his parents used to live, before his father' died and his elderly mother moved to a Moncton apartment.

Two of the three houses on this property were abandoned, the occupants having been unable to go on living here, miles and miles from anywhere.

The patio door slid open and Terry stepped through, carrying two mugs of steaming coffee. We sat, savouring the moment.

This was a tough and lonely place to live. And yet...

'The idea of immersing myself in the blessed silence I've found here appeals.' I realised, as the words left my lips, that the insects were already humming like telegraph wires, though it was not yet nine in the morning.

Terry snorted. 'There's no *blessed silence* here when Don's sawmill is screeching and all the men are in and out, wanting coffee!'

I was glad to have been spared that.

Chapter 9

1.

As we neared Fredericton, we were joined by a large hawk, flying beside Terry's Blazer on my side.

'I've never seen a hawk flying so low!' she exclaimed.

'He came out of nowhere.'

'He's beautiful!'

'Yes.' For several miles, his tawny eye, level with my own, stared back at me as he escorted us into the city.

We reached her brother, Butch's, apartment and knocked on the door. The first thing I noticed was that the man who opened it was rather good looking, with a ready smile and kind eyes, a softer-featured version of Hollywood actor, Michael Douglas.

This was contrary to what I had been led to believe.

'It's too bad my brother's letting himself go,' Terry had mused, sitting above the Salmon River, after the pick-up broke down. 'He's getting fat.'

I had wondered about a blobby brother, when she was so petite herself.

But he wasn't blobby at all.

The hallway was gloomy but wide and long, with several rooms coming off it, so it was a surprise to be led into the bedroom, which seemed an odd place to entertain visitors. It was simply furnished with one single bed and one couch bed on opposite walls, a nightstand, television, computer and closet.

Butch sat on one bed, Terry on the other, beside his sixteen year old son. Mitchel had a shock of strawberry blond hair and a ring in his lip. I sat on a hard-backed chair, between them.

Terry soon launched me into the double act that was evolving as our way of recounting stories:

> T: Then Bobbie said she saw a phone box in the parking lot.
> B: The operator asked for $3.80, so we scrambled around for all our quarters and change.

T: It turned out we had exactly that amount!

B: Pretty much. It took forever to feed the coins into the phone.

T: I told Don we'd broken down. (Deep voice.) "So what do you want me to do?" he said. (Wide-armed shrug.) What do you want me to do?

B: We only had like one minute. I was saying, 'Give him the number of this phone, give him the number of this phone.'

T: So I did. Afterwards, I remembered that you can't receive calls on a public phone in New Brunswick.

B: We were just walking away and it rang.

T: It was Don, calling us on an NB payphone that's not supposed to take incoming calls! Pretty amazing, eh?

We did the same with the deer story, though I backed off when Terry announced that the deer 'came right up to us'. At the next retelling, no doubt, they would be sniffing at our clothing as we petted them.

Terry took Butch out for a private chat. She wanted to get him to buy her boat. That was why we'd tried three times to get here during my stay. While they were gone, Mitchel and I had quite the chat about Soulfest that he had attended with Terry this summer.

He had returned home a Prayer Warrior, unafraid to speak of his beliefs amongst his peers. Such bold commitment to God in one so young was inspirational.

'I heard Tim Hughes sing and play at Soulfest. Do you know him?' he asked. 'He's great. He's from England.'

'Tim Hughes is music director at HTB, my home church!'

'You're from HTB?' He was totally impressed. 'Do you know Nicky Gumbel?'

'He's my vicar!'

'I helped out when my church ran the Alpha Course,' he said. 'I watched him speaking on the Alpha videos.'

'Wow!'

'Wow!'

We grinned at one another. Suddenly, London seemed a lot closer to Canada.

When Terry and Butch returned, I asked whether they had any pets. There was little evidence of Butch and Mitchel's personalities on the white walls and knick-knack free surfaces of this bedroom. I was hoping they'd be pet people.

I was taken into the living room to meet a brown, furry ball in a cage.

'Is it a rat?'

'Chinchilla,' Butch said. 'He's very friendly. You can stroke him.'

Gingerly, I pushed a finger through the bars. Soft cheeks rubbed up against it. What a lonely life the poor creature had in his prison.

'Mitchel, where's Yoshi?' Butch asked.

'Under the couch,' Mitchel replied, crouching down. I crouched down beside him.

As I peered under the couch, Butch crouched down beside me. Though I was looking at the cat, I was pretty sure Butch was looking at my legs. I had on a brown corduroy skirt I had not worn before today because every day at Terry's had been a jeans type of a day.

A pair of startled eyes gleamed as the light caught them. I jumped as, in a nanosecond, the dark outline of a cat morphed into a streak of marmalade that flew towards us and veered away, down the hall.

I knew exactly how Yoshi felt and might have reacted in a similar way to someone eyeing me, before today. But Butch had set the tone for light-hearted flirting as soon as I got here. Within five minutes of my arrival, he had jokingly asked me how I was managing without sex.

To be fair, it was Terry who sparked him off. 'I told her you'd been celibate for three years,' she said.

His sheepish smile was charming. 'Thanks, sis.' He turned to me. 'My marriage ended in divorce, three years ago.'

'It's the same with Bobbie. She's been on her own for two.'

His eyes widened. 'Is that so?' he asked me.

I squirmed with embarrassment. 'Um, yeah.'

'Not so much as a kiss,' Terry assured him, extolling my virtue like a Jewish matchmaker.

He grinned mischievously at me. 'It's tough sleeping alone, isn't it?'

Taken aback by her brother's sauce, I gaped at Terry, who had many times voiced her disapproval of European sexual permissiveness to me. But there would be no help from her, She was smirking, as if such banter were fun. And I found I had to agree. It *was* fun.

I tried to make rising from a squat look effortless. 'Why are we all sitting in the bedroom, when you have this living room?'

It wasn't any more appealing than the bedroom but it had the advantage of being furnished with couches and a coffee table and no beds.

'We share this room with the guys.'

'The guys' turned out to be two residents Butch looked after. This was how he earned his living. Gerry, a short, Down's Syndrome man, clung to me like a long-lost lover when we were introduced. Jamie, whose passion was Ozzy Osbourne, looked somewhat like role model, only a lot bigger. After a mumbled greeting, he shut himself away in his room.

When Gerry completely took over the conversation, I understood why we had initially gone in the bedroom, where Butch and Mitchel could claim some privacy.

Gerry was eager for me to watch him sing so Butch put on a Chris Tomlin CD in Gerry's bedroom, full blast. Gerry grabbed his toy microphone. Flat as a pancake and a beat or two behind, he sang, '*Let God arise! Let God arise!*'

Terry skipped into his room and joined him at the mic.

'*My God reigns now and forever. He reigns now and forever!*' the two of them belted out.

I was in the hallway by the door, dancing and loving it. Butch appeared at my side. 'You love to dance, don't you?'

'Oh, yeah!' I yelled.

'Go in and join them.'

I shook my head, happy out here, with him.

As our visit wound down, I took a photo of Butch, Terry and Mitchel, sitting on Mitchel's sofa bed. Handing Terry my camera, I took her place between them. Butch hesitated for a second before laying an arm across the back of the couch, behind my neck.

At the door, he handed me a scrap of paper with his email and mailing addresses. 'Will you send Mitchel some postcards from London?'

'Yes, I will,' I said.

2.

A bald eagle was circling above Fredericton's spires as we crossed the broad St. John River and drove out of the city. It was a curious place to be hunting, I thought.

'Well, I finally got to meet your brother,' I said.

'Third time lucky,' Terry replied.

I had felt at ease with him. His interest had not seemed a bit predatory. When we sat in a circle to say our parting prayers, he had not been lacking in spirituality, as Terry had hinted. On the contrary, his hand in mine had felt electric.

'That apartment is so dingy. It's depressing,' she said, shaking her head. 'He used to have a big special care home, a beautiful Victorian house with twenty-four residents. It had one of those gorgeous staircases that keeps turning the corner as it goes up, you know?'

I remembered Terry telling me he was a nurturer, like the ravens who fed Elijah. That pleased me. 'What happened?'

'She was unfaithful. He moved out and left her running the business. Not a great decision. With him gone, it kinda fell apart. By the time of the divorce, there was nothing left to divide up.'

'Sad story,' I said.

'Now he's just got two he looks after.'

'Jamie and Gerry.'

'Yeah. I don't know how he does that. I couldn't.'

Neat rows of wooden heritage homes gave way to unpretentious sixties and seventies builds with acreage.

'I don't see him renewing his contract on that apartment,' she said with an air of Terry mystique. 'I see him living in a beautiful house, with trees around it.'

Just like she saw me with a view over water and olive trees, off to the left...

'Today was our last opportunity.' I was glad to have met him, really glad.

'Yes, you're leaving tomorrow.'

'I'm leaving tomorrow.'

We would be continents apart...

'Are you sad?'

'It's been very special.' I was burning to tell her that I liked her brother but I couldn't do it.

I looked back for the eagle but it was nowhere to be seen and the city had melted quite away.

3.

A flock of geese rose from the river as we sped past. Perhaps, like me, they were England-bound. Today was turning out a bird day. It had begun with a pair of finches, 'pulling back the curtains' across our windscreen as we set off this morning. Then came the hawk escort and, finally, the eagle.

The pot-holed roads and ditches had also given us glimpses of porcupines, racoons and skunks.

'My goodness, God's creatures are out in force today!' Terry had cried, as a death-defying mouse scooted across the road, in front of our tyres.

Today, I had felt like we were in a Disney cartoon.

Gradually, neat hayfields and homesteads turned to scrubland and, finally, forest. There was nothing but dark trees and clustering dots of black night, weighing heavily on my eyelids...

I awoke with a start. Terry had said something. 'What is it?'

'The biggest moose you ever saw!'

The windscreen wipers were beating furiously. It was pouring with rain. 'Where?'

The night was black. So was the road.

'Running in the ditch beside us!'

I glimpsed thick antlers, a square snout, a massive, lumbering body.

Tony had warned Terry about the huge moose he and Tia saw near their home. We would be in that area now.

'It's keeping up with us!' In this monochrome world, Terry's face was ghostly white. 'Do I slow down or speed up?'

'I don't know!' Why was she asking me?

After a moment's hesitation, she rammed her foot down hard. We surged forward, leaving the beast, galloping in the ditch behind us.

At the end of a long, tense silence, she let out her breath. 'Phew.'

'I've never seen a moose that close up before!' Come to think of it, I'd probably never seen one at all. It was exciting.

'They run in front of your headlights,' she said, 'and everybody dies.'

4.

That night I dreamt that I was in my house, only it didn't look anything like my real home. The walls were bare and a narrow passage led off a square hallway to the front door. As I stood, boxed-in, the murmur of conversation came to my ears from beyond the living room door, male voices with Canadian accents.

Saddened by the transformation of my house and alarmed by the presence of mystery visitors, I fled to the house of a neighbour, a single woman. I found she had a foreign man of Far Eastern ethnicity in her bed. I was surprised that she had a love life I had not suspected.

I couldn't stay there.

Back at my horrible house again, I could still hear talking. I plucked up the courage to open the living room door and confront these uninvited guests. When I did, however, no one was inside. Like the hallway, this room was pokey and bare, with cracks in the grey, plaster walls.

The bleakness of the dream stayed with me after I awoke. I lay agonising over who I really was, not the lonely woman of my dream, surely? No, I didn't accept that my life was like that.

That woman was more like the one I was before, the one who attended a poetry and dance workshop at London's Laban Centre, a year or so before my marriage ended. When participants were invited to introduce themselves, a Hannah floated to the front and told us that her name meant 'grace', an African woman beat out a rhythm with her foot, but I just stood there, bewildered. Cancer and Seth's abandon had changed me into someone I no longer knew.

Now, however, old things were passed away and I was becoming a new creation in Christ.

'Know what, Bobbie?' Terry had said, sitting on the patio the other morning. 'You look ten years younger than when I was in England last year. You even walk differently and hold your body differently. Now, you look approachable.'

'I was stiff and tight when we were in Israel, too,' I conceded. 'I feel differently now.'

'Your smile sparkles with joy and you radiate peace. It brightens all who see it. I watched my friends react to you at the gathering and it was a pleasure for me to watch.'

'Must be because I'm an Able-Bodied Saviour,' I replied, with a broad grin of pleasure.

I felt I could take on anything with God showing me how to gallop fearlessly into the unknown.

The disappearance of my gold identity bracelet here in Canada seemed to confirm these changes. The bracelet was feminine, with filigree work, made of 22 carat gold and inscribed with, 'Bobbie'. Seth gave it to me, soon after we were married.

It probably fell off somewhere. It may have slipped from my wrist as I walked the shores of Fundy Bay with Terry, Lilly and Heidi on the visit we made to Hopewell Rocks. Or as we sat afterwards, animatedly debating circumcision at the Fundy Bay café, until we realised we might be talking rather loudly.

Its loss spoke of a new ID for me.

Someone, someday, would find my bracelet, perhaps, and, picking away at encrusted red mud, know that 'Bobbie' was once here. But which Bobbie — the one who dreamt she was hemmed in by an ugly house or the one who walked in beauty?

I didn't want to acknowledge that the former even existed. I lay in my bed and took some deep breaths, trying to let God in. An image of the moose behind arrows of rain flashed into my mind. Then those bleak rooms, once again...

I saw myself, drifting through the window on a magic carpet that carried me towards the starry dome outside. I told myself, as I travelled, that I would remember the splendour of this moment when I lay dying, and be comforted.

All at once, black fear draped *itself over my body. It pressed icy fingers to my throat. The* stars are beyond your reach, it mocked, *so where is the comfort in that? There is nothing. All is illusion. The speaking inside of you, the fire of the Holy Spirit — fantasy. God is the ultimate joke.*

A trillion silver pinpricks remained etched upon my lids as I squeezed my eyes tight shut. Tears rolled out of the corners, down towards my ears. I opened them again. Stretching my arm into the molasses night, I unfurled fingers. 'Please.'

5.

'Bobbie, are you awake?'

Wiping away the tears, I fumbled my way through the door and out onto the landing. 'It's 3 am, Terry!'

She stood below me with her hair loose over her shoulders and her dressing gown wrapped around her tiny waist. 'Come down. I've been receiving messages, all about you.'

We sat at the kitchen table, surrounded by pine units that gleamed yellow. Between them, the windows were pitch black holes that made me long for the safety of the yellow glare of suburbia. This house might be hurtling silently through space, suspended in time.

'Don't look so worried, Bobbie. This is for wow tomorrows!'

I assumed she meant an exciting future lay ahead of me. I certainly hoped so after the unnerving dream and darkness I had just experienced.

'I want you to ponder some things that have happened here and seek revelation,' she said. 'Remember that a few days ago, you desired to see a bear, requested to see one? We looked for a bear for a long time — in front, to the sides, up and down tracks, everywhere you'd expect to see a bear. But, as time passed, we realised that there was less and less chance of seeing what we desired to see. We've seen no bear all the time you've been here.'

'Except him,' I said, pointing to the big-headed bearskin on the floor.

'Except him,' she conceded. 'Why was that? Not because the bear wasn't there. It was. Many were. But it wasn't possible to see them, however much you asked. This is profound.'

She'd got me out of bed in the middle of the night to talk in riddles. I stifled a yawn. 'What is?'

'What did we see, Bobbie?' Her fingers rifled her lion's mane. 'Something completely unexpected, a huge moose, running alongside of you. But he didn't hurt you. You should equate this to the unexpected, the moose, unsought, undreamt of, not specifically requested.'

It was too profound for me. I was lost.

She wagged a finger. 'Remember this.'

'Okay.' I pushed back my chair, ready to return to bed, but she had more for me.

'I want to talk to you about the hawk. It was flying in an unexpected place, beside your head, in the same position as the moose, in fact. That was for a reason. When you think of the hawk in the future, you can think of yourself, flying in places you're not supposed to be flying.'

'But I'd like to find where I belong,' I protested, a little fed up of all these predictions that had me on the move. 'I'd like to feel settled.'

She flung her arms wide. 'Your colours will be magnificent. You'll surprise yourself and those around you. Because you're now with the One True Love, you'll be flying places you never thought were possible.'

6.

When Terry eventually released me back to my bed again, sleep continued to elude me.

A procession of creatures passed before my eyes, starting with the deer. Since my experience of New Brunswick wildlife had been one glorious Technicolor movie, I concluded the deer had wanted to show us their babies. What a shame that we had stood there like dummies, when we might have interacted with them, like Cinderella.

I had a flash of insight about Terry's meaning when I got to the moose. She was saying that, though I was asking God for one thing, I would be given another that was equally, if not more, special.

Perhaps my desire for stability was not in His plan. The important thing would be to seize the opportunity He offered. If I didn't do that, the task He had in mind for me might forever remain undone.

I would try to do what God required.

'Lord, if it is your intention to have me running this way and that,' I prayed, 'all I ask of You is to give me the energy, strength and enthusiasm necessary to do it.'

I stretched out my arm again. This time, I reflected that, although I couldn't see my fingers, or even my shoulder, I knew they were there. The night might be black as only somewhere this far from a city could be, but I still believed in my arm, because it was part of me.

7.

Next morning, the sun, streaming in through the bedroom window, warmed the clothes that I was folding and laying in my suitcase, but left me outside of its rays. The starkness of my dream still bothered me. I wanted to lodge a protest that where I was returning to was not like that.

And yet, on one level, I had to admit it was. There was no snow white kitten to cuddle there, nothing and no one. My love life was desolate.

I had had the best twelve days here in New Brunswick. I had realised how much could be achieved in an unstructured way, simply by being available to listen to people. I had begun to explore what it meant to hearten as opportunities presented themselves. I'd loved it.

And I had met a man with laughing eyes, a warm smile, a strong jaw and thick, bronze hair.

I was feeling close to him this morning. How silly was that?

I wanted to marry him.

Where did that idea zing in from? It was sillier still.

But, then again, maybe it was not so far-fetched.

I thought of Ruth who had been so present to me in Israel but had hardly entered my mind since I finished my graphic design course project to lay out the Book of Ruth last May.

When Ruth went out to glean, she 'happened' to pick the field of Boaz, the very man who could save her from her destitution.

What if the explicit purpose of all my signs and wonders had been to lead me here, to meet my Boaz, exactly as God set biblical Ruth up to meet hers, at her moment of greatest need?

Boaz was smitten straight off. He was kind and complimentary. He asked God to bless her. But, once she was done with her gleaning, he seemed to forget her. Weeks went by. In the end, she had to take action herself.

I remembered Terry had told me, sitting above the Salmon River, that, 'My brother's a good guy, but his faith is often more about death than life. Last time I saw him, he told me he couldn't wait to meet his Maker.'

Though he'd appeared cheerful, Butch's gloomy surroundings seemed to support her suggestion that he was depressed. The gentle fragility I detected beneath the cheeky, manly smile had been an attraction to me.

He also hadn't dated for three years.

God had blessed me by putting me in his field but the rest would be up to me. I could see that, if anything was to come of this, I would, like Ruth, have to make the running. .

I could do all things through Christ who strengthened me but could I really pursue a man like she did, risking rejection and humiliation by creeping up to the threshing floor in the middle of the night?

She lay down beside him, which woke him up. He asked her what she wanted.

'Spread your cloak over me,' she said. By that she meant *marry me*.

She was very direct. She wasn't prepared to settle for less. And her tactic worked.

The idea of doing anything like that made me squirm.

Nevertheless, I sent up a prayer: if it was right and it was meant, could it be?

8.

I paused, on my way downstairs, for a last, lingering look at myself on the rug, rope in hand, furrowed brow, hunting down my ibex.

If I could do that, why wouldn't I be flying in places I never thought possible?

I padded on downstairs to the kitchen where Terry was breakfasting on Cheerios.

'I've lost my gold identity bracelet that Seth gave me for my twenty-first birthday,' I told her cheerfully. 'It could be anywhere in New Brunswick. I don't expect I'll ever find it.'

'Oh... dear?' Clearly, she was wondering what I had to smile about.

'I'm okay that it's gone. In fact, it's great. The loss feels like a confirmation that a new me is emerging.'

I was no longer a two-dimensional cut-out, standing in the wings as Terry interacted with people. I was outgoing. I had energy and enthusiasm. I was cheerful. I had compassion for others.

And I was no longer scared of men. I might even be able to find the courage to pursue one.

'Oh, yeah, like a butterfly from a chrysalis,' Terry agreed, beaming.

'Your true self.'

There was a tinge of pride in her voice, as if she considered me her own creation.

And maybe I was, at least to a degree. Her vision had inspired me and her encouragement given me courage.

Without her determination, the two of us would not be here right now.

I had prayed for a man who was kind and a believer and fanciable and Butch fitted the bill on every count. There had been instant chemistry between us. After two years in the wilderness, ducking all advances, a whiff of chemistry was worth its weight in gold.

'By the way' — I ran a finger along the counter, feeling about fourteen — 'I like your brother.'

Her eyebrows shot up. Her spoon wavered in mid-air. She worked at her mouthful. 'Uh, when did this come up for you?'

'When he opened the front door.'

She began to choke. I stepped forward to thump her on the back.

Chapter 10

1.

I reached forward, with a corner of my beautiful, special *tallit* prayer shawl between my fingers, to touch the *Torah* scrolls as they were paraded past me. I then kissed the blue and white threads at the shawl's corner, linking myself in devotion to the Word of God that had been copied out, consonant after consonant, in ornate Hebrew script on yellowing vellum.

Yom Kippur, the Day of Atonement, was always moving and terribly challenging, not simply because we fasted but because we were commanded in the Book of Leviticus to *afflict our souls*. Stepping outside of ourselves to examine our conduct over the past year, admitting our shortcomings and asking for forgiveness could be painful.

Ten days ago, on Jewish New Year, a review of my life began. Today, my fate would be sealed. This was my last chance to lobby God to write me in the Book of Life for a Good Year.

My acceptance of what Jesus did for me on the cross rendered my self-affliction today redundant. Yet, even though He had wiped my slate clean, it seemed good and pleasant to sit together with my brothers and sisters in Judaism and consider where there was room for improvement. I also wanted to give thanks for God's abundant provision.

I said sorry for being Mrs. Angry a lot of the time and sorry for failing to save my marriage. I asked Him for help forgiving those who did me wrong.

On our feet in the synagogue, we made confession together:

We have abused and betrayed. We are cruel.
We have destroyed and embittered other people's lives.
We were false to ourselves.
We have gossiped about others and hated them.
We have insulted and jeered. We have killed. We have lied.
We have misled others...

I was still doing it. I had misled some of my friends, gathered here today, by not being up front about my new faith. I had hidden it away in the pipes, like Snowball hid her kittens, and it was scratching at the ceiling of my conscience.

But, if I told those standing shoulder to shoulder with me now, they wouldn't see me as I saw myself — a completed Jew, in the sense that I believed the longed-for Messiah had come, while they still waited. They would see me as a defector and cancel my synagogue membership. I would no longer receive a ticket to these High Holy Day festivals. I would no longer be welcome at the synagogue. I'd lose my Jewish friends and the entire Jewish community.

The *Torah* scrolls had processed to the altar which, on this solemn Day of Days, was draped in white satin. The rabbi, also dressed in white, was waiting before the scroll cupboard that was framed by white curtains.

Those who had the honour of undressing the scroll he would read from removed the bells, pointer, breastplate, gold-embroidered, white satin sleeve and girdle. Unrolled at the section about to be read, the scroll was lifted high. This was a tricky task that made the man holding it go red in the face as his arms threatened to buckle. Singing in Hebrew, we thanked God for giving us the five books of Moses.

The scroll was laid gently on the altar and the rabbi introduced today's portion, which dealt with the failings of God's people Israel and His enduring love for us, in spite of all.

Even though we read texts about His love, it is my experience that most Jews regard God as Demander of Rigid Obedience. This is particularly true of Orthodox Judaism but is also the case for many Reform and Liberal Jews.

Although Jews have no creed beyond the central command to *Hear O Israel, the Lord our God is One,* (Deuteronomy 6:4), we have 613 *Mitzvot*, or commandments, that control our behaviour. My Reform Synagogue was like synagogues everywhere in respecting these. The more Orthodox synagogues give extra weight to the many rules set by the rabbis in the Oral Law. In many congregations, these are better known and more widely applied than those of *Torah*.

What is sad is how many Jews focus on remembering and observing these rules, yet pay scant attention to loving their neighbour. What I treasured about Jesus' ministry was its message of God's profound fatherly love for us, a love that we should model in our relations with others.

Of course, His message of truth over form rendered Him the natural enemy of those Jews who were sticklers for the letter of the Law in His own time.

If Jews preoccupied with form tended to miss out on a close relationship with a loving God, I had noticed in my short time as a Believer that many Christians missed out on the richness of the context of Jesus.

Almost everything He, or anyone else in the New Testament, said or did referenced the traditions, sayings and prophecies of the Old Testament that was dear to me. They confirmed Jesus as the fulfilment of God's purposes since the Creation.

Even though He was Perfect and had nothing to atone for, He was standing beside me now in this synagogue, listening to the rabbi reading from the scroll — and wincing a little, perhaps, because his Hebrew was bad enough for even a beginner like myself to flinch at it.

Every year, Jesus would have made *Yom Kippur*, just as He kept all the other Jewish festivals.

On the cross, He became our *Kippur*, our atonement. He was both the goat that was sacrificed for our sins and the scapegoat that was released to carry them away, into the wilderness, a tradition still upheld by some Jews today.

I got it that, by going to the cross during Passover, Jesus linked *Kippur* to *Pesach* and became all things to us. He became our Pardon, our Sacrifice and also our Saviour — the Pascal Lamb of the Exodus, whose daubed blood saved the Israelite slaves to life when the Angel of Death passed over them.

At the Passover *Seder*, my family and Jews everywhere tell the story of how God brought Moses and the Children of Israel to freedom in the Promised Land. The Last Supper was the Passover *Seder* meal, after which Jesus announced that He was about to lead God's children into the Promised Land of Eternal Life.

He made *kidush* and *hamotzi* — He broke bread and they shared it and blessed a cup of wine from which all present drank, just as I did in my home to welcome in the Sabbath and the Festivals. The difference was that Jesus was symbolically sanctifying His broken body and spilled blood of which all could partake, so long as they did it in remembrance of Him.

At this time, He spoke to his disciples of the New Covenant, foretold by the prophet Jeremiah, through which God confirmed His new, personal relationship with us: He would live in my heart, rather than on tablets of stone.

As Moses descended with these tablets from the mountain at Pentecost, Jesus ascended to Heaven, to prepare a place for me in the new Promised Land.

Though I loved the solemnity of this *Kippur* day, I could never step backwards to distance and rigidity again. God's smile on my face in the morning was like a kiss. All day long, His Holy Spirit was a warm place inside of me.

2.

I did not have the *chutzpah* to write directly to Butch. I wrote to his son, Mitchel. After all, Butch had asked me to do that.

I wrote that I'd soon be sending him the postcards of London his Dad told me he wanted...

My fingers hovered above the keyboard. I gazed out of my study window. The summer was over. Leaves were congregating in the middle of the road to hurl themselves down the street in a September Uprising.

I touched briefly on the autumn shop windows at Harrods that I passed on my way to worship at HTB and when I went to help out with the Divorce and Separation Recovery Course.

I mentioned the colours of the trees in Hyde Park...

Remembering that he was a bright kid, strong in the Lord, I described *Yom Kippur* at the synagogue and some of my feelings about that.

With best wishes, Bobbie

3.

I had to be up early in the morning.

I should have gone straight to bed when I got in from my Jewish friend's party: giggles and great fun over dinner at her house, toasts to the bride, for she would soon be getting married.

Instead, I sat at my desk and opened up my computer.

The heating was purring, now that the nights had turned chilly. My house was full of creaks and sighing joists.

Three days had passed and there had been no word from Canada. I guessed that was the end of it. Never mind, I supposed. I trusted that God would open those doors that were meant to open for me.

A new message was in my Inbox. I opened it. The reply was from the father, not the son. Butch didn't have a lot to say for himself: the weather in Fredericton was sunny, Mitchel was doing well at school... But it was a nibble and that was what counted.

4.

'You see, Bobbie,' Alicia told me, 'when I was a kid, Jews for Jesus would hang about the streets of Toronto in order to strike up conversations with unsuspecting Jews. They would then try to break chains of faith and Jewish identity that had been handed down from generation to generation, for thousands of years.'

She had come to see me to explain why she and my son, Jeremy, found it so difficult to accept my switch to Christianity. More specifically, she wanted me to understand why he wasn't prepared to keep the diary with devotions I bought him at the bible bookstore in Moncton where Terry's friend, Lilly, worked.

Though the return of the diary hurt me, since it was a snub, I sort of understood. Veronica's conviction that her Christian beliefs were right and better than my Jewish ones used to make me fume.

But I also now understood that Jesus said, 'No one comes to the Father except through me.'

I offered Alicia tea or coffee but it was clearly not that kind of a visit. When we hung out as family at the weekends, it was almost always at their place, where my granddaughters had all their toys and videos and dressing up clothes and books and games.

'Neither of us wants Christian books in the house,' she explained in a tone that was firm but loving.

Jeremy and Alicia liked to keep the Jewish festivals at home. They were members of the same Reform synagogue I was, although they never attended Saturday worship, as I had been in the habit of doing, until recently. However, my two granddaughters attended the Sunday morning religion school.

'And I'm returning the olive branch refrigerator magnets, as well.' She laid them on the coffee table, pretty ceramics, with painted motifs.

I stared at them and tried to mask the feelings of rejection welling up. 'They represent Israel,' I said, not knowing how else to argue in their favour.

Jeremy and Alicia were very pro-Israel.

'They're from the Christian Mission to the Jews,' she said. 'That's a missionary organisation.'

She said 'missionary' as if the word tasted bad.

I wanted my family to share in the loving God I had found. To keep the truth to myself would be to deprive them. But they didn't want to hear, neither Jeremy and Alicia, nor Simon and Sylwia, when I visited them down in Cornwall, nor Tania who was training to be a maths teacher at a boarding school near Birmingham.

I felt more alone in my house than I'd felt in a long time, after Alicia left.

5.

I discovered Butch had three children, two boys and a girl, the same as me. Mitchel was his youngest.

The emails grew longer, stuff about what we did, what we liked and what we thought, confirmation that we were in one another's prayers.

To Butch:

This time last year, when Terry visited me in England, I was full of bitterness for my broken marriage. Somehow, though, I've come to accept that I couldn't live with the little that was on offer. That was my choice. And it's okay.

Do you plan to come to England at any stage?

To Bobbie:

Not at the present time. I live my days looking a few years ahead constantly.

He was scrimping and saving.

To Butch:

Are your days all stuff to be got through?

To Bobbie:

I do make the choice to remain positive and cheerful. It makes those around you so much happier. I've made wrong choices in life and have paid the price but know that, with solid planning and God's help, things will turn around.

The decision to leave his former wife in charge of their special care home had left him broke, though he was back on his feet and solvent now, with a steady income from the Province for looking after his two residents.

To Butch:

I would like your days to be good days, not just where you tell yourself they're good and smile. I will pray for you to have good days.

6.

Deep in the Spirit, I responded to an invitation to come forward for prayer at the Daughters of the King women's conference.

'There's a rug,' I told Debbie, the softly-spoken, young keynote speaker. 'It's a rug of prophecy and I don't understand it. Could you pray for some clarity?'

She smiled and placed a hand on my shoulder.

I was in a beautiful space, both in my head and physically. This contemporary, South London, Anglican church, with clean lines of brick and pine, was pleasing.

Debbie's beauty lay in the way she glowed. As she began to pray, whispering beneath her breath at first and then asking for more, all my old surgical scars began to ache. Parts of me that were numb were coming back to life again, just like in the Prayer Tower in Jerusalem.

Eventually, she opened her eyes and said slowly, 'This is what is coming to me. It's about careful weaving, it's about adjustments and planning and laying it out and trying it, until it looks as it's meant to look. It's about creating from love and sticking with it, until it's right. It's expressing the seasons. And it's not finished.'

Her words left me bemused. She had spoken as if I were the weaver.

7.

I relayed this and further details of my special day to Butch, via email.

I was given a verse, written out on a scroll. They had prayed for me when I signed up for the women's day and come up with a verse from Isaiah: This is my chosen one, in whom I delight.

I found that beautiful.

There was some mistake. I was given the same scroll twice. Everyone received a different scroll but I was the only one who received two scrolls and they were identical. That felt extra special.

Later, in the afternoon, we were invited forward to pick stones from a 'stream' of blue cloth, draped on the ground. The stone I chose said 'teacher' on the reverse. That pleased me, too.

Much food for thought here. I don't know what, to whom, where or by what method I will teach. Not yet, at least. But I really like the idea.

I remembered that Bero had asked me whether I was a teacher...

To Bobbie:

It sounds as though the Lord has plans for you as a teacher. I think you could be an effective teacher in whichever direction you were to go.

'But he takes several days to reply each time,' I grumbled to Terry over the phone. 'Is he really interested?'

'He's typing with two fingers,' she said 'Anything more than a sentence is a real compliment to you.'

After a little hesitation, she had decided she was all in favour of this budding relationship with her brother. She was seeing a lot of him herself these days, visiting him frequently and even staying over.

Our own conversations had grown less frequent and less intense. We hardly discussed the rug any more. What she mainly wanted to do was rant about Don, who couldn't be pinned down to discussing their problems, she said.

When I asked Butch about happiness, he wrote:

To Bobbie:

I was always happy when I was holding a baby. I've found periods during my life when I was financially secure that I enjoyed life much more than was possible when I wasn't. I've fond memories of travel, fishing, skydiving... It seems I've spent too much time planning happiness for the future, but just lived day-to-day.

A picture was emerging of a man who was patient and loved children. I could tell from how Mitchel had turned out that he had been a good dad. This was also a man who looked at himself and tried to put right mistakes.

Can I ask you the same question?

I gave a lot of thought to my reply:

To Butch:

When I had cancer, four of us were friends together. Two are now dead and one has a recurrence. Sometimes that makes me wobbly and vulnerable but mostly I celebrate. I rejoice in every extra sunset God gives me.

Strangely, my best happy moment comes from that miserable time in the depths of chemotherapy.

It was a Saturday evening and, rather than watch tv, my children ended up flopped on my big bed. I was too poorly to really say much but they were on fine form, chatting and joking together. I just loved being there, looking at the great people they had become, and I knew myself happy.

8.

Terry was back from yet another visit to Butch. I envied her.

'He was sitting at his computer in the bedroom as I went in,' she told me on the phone. 'On the screen was a photo of you and Tania! *Hey, that's Bobbie's daughter!* I cried. *Yes*, he said, *Bobbie sent me some photos of her weekend visiting her daughter.* It's something else when I have to go all the way to Fredericton to catch up on *my* best friend's news!'

Though I laughed at her mock outrage, I didn't tell her we now emailed daily. I thought she might get genuinely peeved at that.

'He said you guys went horseback riding?'

'Yeah, Tania rode her horse, Kettle, and I borrowed someone else's.'

I had hardly ridden since I had to have Dizzy put down.

Dizzy was the beautiful thoroughbred horse I bought to mark my survival from cancer. He had turned out to have health problems of his own. One day, for no apparent reason, he morphed into a rodeo horse, throwing me violently enough to put me in a wheelchair for a while.

Though my broken hip eventually got better, sadly my bucking bronco did not. A veterinary investigation into the causes of his behaviour revealed a painful equine condition called kissing spine.

There was no telling when he might go crazy again so I couldn't sell him on. Neither could I put a fancy pants horse like he was out to grass, where he would surely wither away.

Regretfully, I took the decision to lead him out to the muck heap one grey, English morning. There the knacker put a pistol to his blaze that was shaped like a back-to-front question mark. The sound of the shot rolled around the meadows as he went down and all the birds took to the air.

'Butch said you hadn't been on a horse in five years.'

'That's right.'

With the risk of haemorrhage from the blood-thinning medication I was prescribed for the lung clots that succeeded the broken hip, I was afraid I might bleed to death if I fell off again. In any case, I was lukewarm about riding school dobbins and done with having a horse of my own.

'So how did you like it?'

'I was nervous at first, but it soon got so I was loving being out, loving that high-up perspective on the world. But I can hardly walk now.'

It had been three days and I was still hobbling. Every muscle ached and my skeleton felt like someone had shaken it.

'He took me through *all* the photos you sent *him*.' Her tone implied this was a long process.

'A few shots of my weekend with Tania,' I protested, not wanting her to feel left out.

'There was one of the two of you, standing either side of a horse at the stable door.'

'*Wow, she's beautiful*! Butch said. I leaned in for a closer look and said, *Yes, her eyes are gorgeous, a really unique shade of turquoise.* He looked at me like I was from a different planet. *They're brown!* he said,

Oh, you mean the daughter! Never mind the daughter. Look at the mother!'

I giggled. I felt coy and pleased at the same time.

'His expression was as dumb as that goofy horse. By the sound of it, so is yours, right now.'

9.

To Bobbie:

What do you have planned for the weekend?

I guessed he had no plans.

To Butch:

You asked me about my weekend. Lots going on – family breakfast at Jeremy and Alicia's tomorrow, craft fair in the afternoon, meeting of HTB's Creativity and Arts Group on Sunday and staying for the 5 pm service after.

My life seems to be very busy. It's not what I want all the time. My perfect weekend would be much more like a slow-moving river.

I was thinking of the deep blue Salmon River, where Terry and I had sat when the pick-up broke down, enjoying the sunshine and conversation in surroundings removed from the world.

What would yours be?

To Bobbie:

It sounds like you're going to be very busy. I find my daily routine of caring for Jerry and Jamie and Mitchel about the extent of my activities.

A weekend spent like a slow-moving river sounds like something to enjoy.

Thank you for being interested in my life. You are a good friend.

Chapter 11

1.

I had it in my mind to get good at visual design and link that to my writing. Continuing with the range of arts courses I was signing up for that, so far, had included sketching and fantasy picture making, as well as narrative illustration and my certificate in graphic design, for which I had gained a merit, I was now taking the Textiles Course at London's City Lit.

The theme for the autumn term's project was 'Treasure'. I chose to depict the Good Woman from Proverbs 31, whose worth was far above rubies.

I had long loved the bible's description of this businesswoman who worked with wool and flax and was like the merchant ships, bringing food from afar. She bought a field and planted a vineyard, she made tapestry and linen garments and sashes and sold them. She perceived that her merchandise was good. Her lamp did not go out at night.

She was practical and righteous and strong. She opened her mouth in wisdom and on her tongue was the law of kindness. Above all, she was treasured by her husband and family.

Any kind of comprehensive image of this woman would be too diffuse, I decided, for her life was so full and varied. My picture would be stronger if I homed in on just one of her twenty-two attributes, (one for every letter of the Hebrew alphabet, in sequence).

My choice: *She does not fear the snow for her household*, was an odd one that I could not readily explain to myself. I told my teacher that I thought it would be interesting and challenging to work with the blues and pinks and pale greys of the snow pallet, rather than the bold reds, golds and oranges I usually preferred.

It was only as my textile picture began to take shape that I realised that the subject was inspired by a vision of virgin snow I once had. About to leave the marital home, I had sat quietly and asked to be shown what my life would become. Slowly, a picture had come together before me, a broad field of virgin snow, rimmed by fir tres.

There had been nothing else, no animals or birdsong, just a place of pristine beauty, white and cold.

This landscape was frightening but also beguiling. Something told me the snow was deep. I might stumble or disappear without trace in the drifts, suffocated by the cold snow. Yet the prospect of making footprints excited me.

I had noted the vision down in my diary and hardly thought any more of it. Going back to check it out released the same feelings of expectancy and fear as before.

I realised that what I wanted to express today through a picture entitled She Does Not Fear The Snow was how it felt to trust in God and allow Him to lead me.

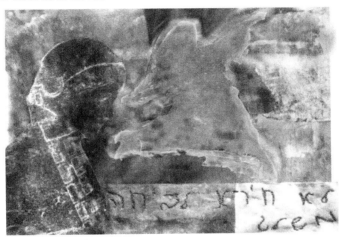

The result of my art project was a lot dreamier than my usual work. The Good Woman stood in profiled silhouette of gleaming bronze before hazy images of Jerusalem, under snow. At the same time, she danced across the centre of the picture, swathed in mauves and blues.

I was pleased with how it turned out.

2.

Butch calling me a good friend spurred me on to up the ante:

You've told me I'm a good friend. I hope we are now firm friends but it would be good to have the opportunity to explore whether there could be more. Do you agree? (It's okay to say not.)

I was confused by the reply I received.

We are definitely firm friends. I'd love to explore whether there could be more at some point. It's going to take a couple of years of personal sacrifice to be in the position to have enough freedom to enjoy more. I'm flattered. You're a beautiful woman.

3.

I watched, fascinated, as strands of spaghetti writhed like worms at the end of my friend, Valerie's, fork. 'He says you're a beautiful woman.'

I glanced nervously around me. I didn't want everyone in this trendy restaurant — mirrored walls, steel chairs, blue and black decor —to know that I, a mature woman of fifty-five, was in a quandary about dating. 'But, *I'd love to explore whether there could be more at some point*?'

'Eh?'

'It sounds like a put-off.'

'Read it again,' she said.

I had the email with me. '*It's going to take a couple of years of personal sacrifice to be in the position to have enough freedom to enjoy more. I'm flattered. You're a beautiful woman.* See?'

I gazed down at my half-finished risotto and heaved a sigh, my appetite gone.

Valerie was not about to allow me to wallow in self-pity. 'Put yourself in his place, Bobbie. He's been on his own, not so much as dating, for three whole years. That's a long time.'

'Tell me about it.' Two was more than long enough.

'He's smitten but feeling inadequate.' Her heart-shaped face, rimmed by a dark bob, tilted this way and that as she warmed to her subject. 'He was once successful but now he's somewhat strapped for funds. He's wondering: What can I possibly offer any woman, let alone an exciting, beautiful, international woman like her, she doesn't already have?'

I was embarrassed by her compliments but got what she was saying. And I knew the answer. 'Love, kindness, time together,' I said.

'He's thinking: Give me time to save some pennies. Then I might feel differently.'

'A hundred years ago, when I was last on the market, it was a lot easier than this.'

Her sharp blue eyes narrowed. 'It wasn't. You've forgotten.'

'No, you've forgotten. You've been happily married forever. He's saying thanks but no thanks.'

'I don't think so.'

'You really don't?'

'He's saying he'd like to take things forward,' she said, 'But can't because of his circumstances.'

'Do you think?'

4.

There was a good-looking, single man of my age at HTB's Creativity and Arts Group the next Sunday. An actor showed us how to read expressively from the Bible and we practised extracts from the Christmas story. Afterwards, we all went into the 5 o'clock worship service together.

I couldn't say whether this man was interested in me or not. I detected no spark. But then, I gave him zero encouragement.

I realised, as the Circle Line tube train shunted me left and right, that I'd started saving myself for Butch.

This was becoming silly.

I had met this man only once. His response to my enquiry about a possible relationship was that he would be ready in about two years.

I'd had cancer. I might not have two years.

I wrote him an email as soon as I got home. It said:

About exploring what might be. Thank you for the lovely things you said. It'd be good to go for a walk, have a cup of coffee, share a meal. We might very quickly say, 'Oh, no, this is not right!' But knowing that would be almost as valuable as knowing the opposite, for it takes us forward in our lives. I suppose one of us has to travel 3,000 miles to find that out. I think what you're saying is the one has to be me?

I rang Valerie, ready to justify my actions.

I didn't need to. She heartily approved. 'It's good you're going there. It puts you in control. If it's a disaster, you can hop on a plane to New York and do some shopping.'

She was the one who loved New York. That would not be my kind of thing but I accepted the sentiment. 'He could still email me that he's too busy, or not reply at all!'

'No way, Bobbie.'

The phone was ringing. Valerie probably had something she'd forgotten to say...

But it was a North American male voice that said, 'Hi.'

'Hi.'

'It's me, Butch.'

Though this looked like a delightful result, my heart began to thud. I wondered if he could hear it.

'I know.'

Oh no, I sounded as bashful as a three-year-old in front of Father Christmas.

'How are you today?'

'Good.' I was as fidgety as a three-year, too. In the bedroom, squirmed down onto my back on the carpet and hooked my ankles over the radiator under the window sill. I had never in my life conducted a phone conversation in this position.

Since the radiator was burning hot, I had to knead my feet like a kitten.

'Hi.'

'Hi.'

'So you'd like to come visit?' His voice was so deep.

'Yeah.' My face was hotter than my feet. 'I'll stay at a hotel. How far is the Ramada from you?'

(Derr, how uncool, letting him know I'd gone into that already!)

'Not far. When will you come?'

'I don't know.' I doodled figures of eight across the radiator's surface with my roasted feet. 'When would you like?'

'Tomorrow?'

'Tomorrow!'

Whoa, he'd been transformed from Mr. Cool into Mr. Keen.

I shunted around to sit, cross-legged. 'I could make it in two or three weeks, maybe.'

I had things to do, not the least of which was get used to the idea of going on a date.

5.

Terry hijacked the conversation when I called to tell her that I was coming to Fredericton.

'We're going to be taking care of people during a time of great crisis,' she said. 'We're going to be ministering to the Jews first and then the Gentiles. You are to learn Israeli Hebrew, because it's going to be mainly Jews you'll be ministering to and many will be in Israel.'

A lot of Terry's prophecies had turned out to be accurate. But not all of them. I reserved judgement on this latest assertion, delivered in a tone that implied she expected me to jump up and take part in the action.

'We're in an army,' she said. 'That's why we're on horses.'

I expressed my misgivings by a silence she did not even seem to notice. What she was saying and the way she was now saying it concerned me. I thought Terry probably needed to sleep. She didn't sleep much when we were in Israel, back in March. At her home last month, she had been up nearly every night.

But I could not tell her that. There was no telling her anything.

'More clarity is coming, every day,' she went on. 'We have to see that no impure thing touches us. Seek purity.'

Though I remembered that she was told, 'Purity is the key,' at Soulfest, I didn't know what she meant.

I said. 'When I pray, it seems God is telling me that many people will try to define our mission according to their own inclinations.'

I meant her but she didn't understand.

'That's right, Bobbie.'

A few nights later, the phone woke me in the middle of the night. I couldn't get to answer it in time. In my fuzzy state, I heard Terry's voice, leaving a long and rambling message on my machine. 'I have been given clarity, Bobbie. God is angry. He's sending a storm, a terrible and devastating storm. There will be deaths. Many will be injured. He is going to punish the sin in the City of Moncton, wipe it right out. The sinners should repent now. It will happen Thursday.'

She had stepped over a line. She had gone from receiving prophecies to seeing herself as a prophet.

6.

HTB was an hour away, in Central London. When I couldn't get there for worship, I sometimes attended another charismatic, Anglican church nearer home, Christchurch in Anerley. This was the church that hosted the Daughters of the King Conference, where the keynote speaker had seen me as the weaver of the rug.

This church had a heart for Israel and the Jews. At *Sukkot*, the Jewish festival of Tabernacles, I had helped build a *sukkah* in the sanctuary, decorating a makeshift shelter with fragrant fruit and green branches.

On this particular Sunday morning, I was deep in prayer, thinking about Jesus' call to the thirsty in the Temple during that festival. He was likening Himself to the Great Altar, which was repeatedly drenched in living water by the High Priest, throughout *Sukkot*. The image of Jesus as a source of abundant water was a powerful one, in a parched land like Israel.

A sense of movement around me brought me back to the present, though I still jumped when I opened my eyes to see a man and a woman, standing right in front of me, with their hands outstretched over me.

'God loves you,' the woman said. She was tall, taller than her husband. They were both of retirement age. 'He knows your specialness and your worth.'

The man's speech was strange. He had suffered a stroke and could not get his sentences out. The words came in a jumble. 'For your faith all faiths... here not just...'

He broke off, embarrassed.

'Go on, please,' I said. I wanted to take away any pressure he felt to speak quickly. I also wanted to hear what he had to say.

'Here not just, not this church... but everywhere... Everybody for... the whole world.' He frowned, frustrated with himself.

'My faith is universal?'

He squeezed my hand in his.

I liked what he had said very much.

7.

To Butch:

'I've been having long chats with God about what to pray for regarding this trip but, this morning, I hit upon a request for Him to just bless every aspect of it.'

To Bobbie:

'I will pray that the Lord bless every aspect of your trip. I feel that I've already been blessed to have you as a friend. I'm really looking forward to getting to know you better. We will feel much more comfortable talking after this visit. We've already discussed some pretty intense things.

We had both explained what happened to our marriages.

I do realise that, in order for us to truly know one another, the past must be clear.'

8.

The topic of moving on and building new lives with new partners came around again at the Divorce and Separation Recovery Course, which I was now helping to facilitate.

In the hopes of giving a boost to the two lovely women in my small group who had no self-confidence and didn't believe that they would ever fall in love again, I decided to share what was going on in my own life.

'When it was my turn to talk about dating as a participant on this course, six months ago, I expressed a desire for something I thought didn't exist. I wanted a deep and meaningful relationship straight off, without all the posturing and trying to impress that goes with starting-out relationships. And this is what God has granted me,' I told them. 'I have yet to go on a first date and already we know one another well. Already I feel as if we're falling in love.'

9.

Veronica's mouth was a rectangle of tangled emotions as she leaned across my coffee table. Her compassion for me pained her, she had her mind set on setting me straight and she was indignant about my misguided choices. 'Do you really think it wise to consider such a man?'

I was sorry now to have even mentioned Butch.

'He's been married before, you say?'

'Yes.'

'What happened?'

'The wife was unfaithful.'

Her eyebrows knitted. 'Perhaps the husband neglected her!'

I had to smile because it sounded as if she was justifying conduct that she would have condemned in anyone else.

'He's a PK, Veronica, a preacher's kid. His Dad was a Baptist Minister. He's always tried to be upstanding before God, so he married the woman he took up with, when perhaps he shouldn't have.' Looking her straight in the eye, I said, 'I can shy away from him because of the label he's wearing, or I can find out for myself what he's like.'

'But, Bobbie, you're giving this man the kind of chance you wouldn't give Seth!' She was as scrappy as a terrier in her fight for my soul.

Self-righteous exasperation balled in my stomach. I just about managed to keep my voice level. 'Seth wants to do as he pleases. It's been very hard but I've accepted it. Why can't you?'

She clicked her tongue. 'Because it may still not be too late for his eyes to be opened!'

'Look, Veronica, since I left two years ago, there's been no turning towards me, no desire. The one date we had, which was a disaster, was as a result of my calling him.'

'It's not about desire,' she said. 'It's about obedience. The Lord wants you to stay with your husband.'

With a flash of insight, I realised how my claim to freedom rocked her own boat, for it called into question her decision to stick with her husband, whose commitment to Judaism led him to deplore the Christianity she had embraced.

Her big dream was to win him over and lead him to faith. It was vital to her that I should do all I possibly could to try and achieve the same with Seth. If God were to bless me in any other course of action, what would that imply for her choices?

I picked up my mug of coffee and took a sip. 'The Lord can't want me to stay with Seth,' I said, 'because He doesn't ask of us what we cannot do and I can't do that.'

10.

I asked Valerie to come and reassure me.

'Look at what I'm doing, chasing half way across the world after a man I've met only once!'

We were in my living room with the gas log fire cosy and throws over our knees, sipping the wine she had brought.

She tilted her head. 'What links you?'

'He's a storm chaser. He loves nature and walks. We like good food. We might cook together.'

None of this was anything Butch and I had actually done together. I felt like I was selling her on an idea.

Nonetheless, I could see her ticking off the boxes on her mental checklist. 'You have quite a lot in common, then.'

'And we both love the Lord.' I still felt a little awkward using pious expressions like this. Valerie believed in God but led a secular life.

She took a sip from her glass and nodded. 'That, too.'

'I think I could live in Canada,' I said and laughed. 'I feel so weird, talking that way.'

Valerie was ever practical. 'There'd be no point in going, if you weren't prepared to follow through on it.'

'Of course, we could end up in the UK.'

All that would need to be decided as the need arose, I supposed.

'I love how up-front Butch is when he doesn't know stuff.' I was on firmer ground here, talking from experience of our phone calls and emails. 'He doesn't seem to resent it or feel threatened if I know stuff. But he has no academic qualifications.'

Now I sounded like I was checking him over like I a horse, weighing up the positives and negatives ahead of deciding whether or not to buy. And perhaps that was what I was doing.

'Neither does Matthew.'

'Right.' I had forgotten that because I always thought of her husband as someone who was very wise. Yet she was the one with the Masters, while he had had little formal education. I was pleased to hear it and felt reassured.

The CD changed and Eva Cassidy filled the room. Conversation fell away. Valerie looked at me searchingly. I grinned back, knowing that she had seen straight through to the scaredy cat inside.

'Bobbie, you need to actually put yourself there, in an intimate situation.'

I smiled on, though a pair of tongs had gripped my heart. I couldn't put myself there at all. 'That may not happen.'

'But it might,' she insisted. 'You're a beautiful woman. You're sexy, inwardly and outwardly.'

I forced a laugh. 'I don't feel sexy.'

Yet, these last few days, my body seemed to have been coming out of hibernation. There had been strange tinglings and the wish to be held so strong it made me cry. I had never felt this way before.

It terrified me.

'Does he know?' she asked.

Oh dear, I was in danger of crying. 'He knows I've had a...' I pointed at my reconstructed breast. '...er, cancer.'

This was a different, kinder man. I had dreamed he stood, holding my hand as I slept, and I had felt safe. This man would be healing. He wouldn't push me away or cast me off.

'He doesn't know... I haven't told him... that I look like I've been in a bad accident.'

There was no holding back the tears now. They were rolling down my cheeks.

'There's more to you than a boob,' Valerie asserted.

I shook my head. 'So much of who Seth and I were turned out to hinge on my breasts.'

She was indignant. 'Any man who'd consider that important isn't worth it.'

I didn't trust my voice to answer her.

She became practical. 'Do you have a negligee, some pretty undies?'

'Um, I don't think...'

'Plain white cotton won't work. Do you have something to make you feel really feminine? You don't, do you?'

'Um....'

11.

To Butch:

'I dare say you're nervous too. Don't worry about filling up my time.

I'm very self-contained.

To Bobbie:

I'm glad you're coming to visit. It will be good to spend time with you and have the opportunity to become closer friends. There's really no down side to your visit. Don't allow yourself to feel nervous, I'm not.

Of course he was nervous. At least that was what a friend's husband maintained. He said guys just liked to pretend they're not nervous.

Before taking the giant leap of faith of going up to the threshing floor, Ruth gave herself a boost by immersing herself in the purifying waters of the *mikvah*, rubbing perfumed oils into her skin and putting on freshly-laundered clothing. I got a new skirt, a colour and cut, a manicure and a facial.

I crept out in the dark, like Ruth, for my early morning flight. As well as the usual clot preventative measures, I needed plenty of prayer to carry me through the mega, eight-hour flight to Toronto, and the further two, back to Fredericton.

Chapter 12

1.

Butch stopped the car outside my hotel.

'It's been a great day,' I told him.

'I wanted to put my arm around you at the apartment,' he said, 'but I was shy.'

He was showing restraint and giving me my space physically, for which I was grateful. The last thing I wanted was to feel under pressure.

He backed the car a few feet, away from the welcoming lights of reception, and leaned towards me for our first kiss. He knew how to kiss.

I clung to him with my head resting on his chest, listening to the thud-thud of his heart. 'I really like you.'

'I know you do.' He paused, teasing me with silence, before adding, 'I really like you, too.'

He drove the car forward again, onto the drop-off ramp.

'Goodnight,' I said.

'Goodnight.'

I got out of the car and waved as I went through the doors to the foyer, trying to look casual on the outside, inwardly restraining myself from punching the air.

All through the long journey here, I had been wondering whether I was in for a big let-down at Fredericton airport. But, as soon as I saw him, I knew I had been right to come.

I was dreading awkward hellos with a bunch of flowers, but he brought along Mitchel and Down's Syndrome resident, Gerry, to normalise the contrived situation, and saved the flowers — red and yellow roses and a basket of fruit and chocolates — for me to find in the privacy of my hotel room.

I stole sidelong glances as we waited for my suitcase, checking whether he was as fanciable as I remembered. He was.

After a short search for Gerry, who was trying to board a flight with my used boarding pass, we poured out into the chilly, New

Brunswick night and headed for my hotel. Butch dropped me there, so I could freshen up, and returned for me later, alone.

We parked by the St. John River, across from Fredericton's pretty city lights, and talked. I do not remember what we said — it was about 2 a.m. in my head and my ears felt like cotton wool from the whirring propeller plane — but I found his melodic voice a delight.

In the days that followed, we went for drives beneath puddle-grey skies, along riverbanks rimed with frost. Snow-dusted trees struck convoluted poses as we flashed by, discussing beauty and the bible and abortion and American politics. We sat in Starbucks and talked some more. I found him easy, genuine and frank.

We got on so well that spending even part of our days apart was not an option.

At the apartment, we sat in the kitchen with Mitchel, Gerry and his other resident, Jamie, who referred to me as 'Butch's woman', until Butch pointed out that he shouldn't say that.

Gerry squinted at me in his endearing way and called me his 'little cupcake'.

'Back off, Gerry,' Butch warned. 'She's mine, not yours.'

His tone was jokey but I was happy to hear him say this. We had communicated so much before this visit that I felt like I knew him already. I had needed to verify that the attraction I thought I'd felt at that first meeting was real. It was. Even though the strangeness of dating a man still left me ill at ease, I felt like I was his.

Gerry looked thoughtful. 'Maybe I could marry Jamie.'

Jamie, hunched over the table, rolling cigarette after cigarette, only grinned.

'You can't marry, Jamie,' Mitchel said. 'He's a man.'

'But I'd like to get married.' Gerry looked downcast but only momentarily. 'I know, I'll dress up as Mrs. Doubtfire. Then we can get married!'

We all laughed.

Pleased with himself, Gerry tweaked an imaginary bow tie. 'Good idea!'

In a house filled with men, I became a female curiosity. Michael, Butch's elder son, dropped by and told me I had daunting eyes. (To this day, I do not know what he meant by that.) The trainers I took off in the hallway were examined and discussed. The socks I was wearing were noticed and commented upon. They seemed to receive everyone's approbation.

2.

Another day spent together. Another goodnight kiss in the parking lot.

The days were passing.

Back in my hotel room, I alternated between pacing the floor and sitting in the armchair by the desk, staring at the pretty roses and basket of fruit Butch gave me. I wasn't ready to get into bed.

Dear God, please continue to bless every aspect of this trip.

Butch was leaving me the lead in taking our relationship to another level. I didn't like it anymore. Was I going to have to go up to the threshing floor at night, uncover his feet and lay down, to claim him?

The woman in me wanted to do that. The screwed-up cancer survivor didn't dare.

A memory had been playing over and over in my mind, like an old record stuck in the groove: Seth, on the phone, congratulating Terry on little Lonnie's birth and telling her to work on getting her figure back.

'Remember,' he sniggered, 'Men don't like their women straight up and down.'

I was sitting right beside him, straight up and down from the mastectomy, about to go into hospital for the breast reconstruction surgery that would fail miserably and nearly cost me my life.

My battle to rebuild myself would continue. Eventually, I had to accept that a sundae of silicone implant and *latismus dorsi*, with a twist of flesh on top to replicate a nipple, was going to be the very best I could achieve.

If Butch so much as averted his eyes, I'd be a cowering wreck forever.

Seeking encouragement, I phoned my Naomi. 'Terry, what should I do? He's being respectful.'

She started to tell me at length how she came to her first marriage a virgin. I was glad to note that she was sounding a lot more cheerful than in the last few weeks.

She had initially called the devastating storm she was predicting for Thursday, then Friday, the weekend... Monday... and holed herself up in the basement with provisions. Taking Lonnie downstairs with her had tipped the balance for Don. What happened next was unclear.

I'd spoken to both on the phone. He was bewildered. She was furious.

A major storm had come, just as Terry had prophesied, but it had been in their lives only. Their marriage was in deep crisis.

'Just a second,' I cut in. This was, after all, long distance from my hotel room on my dime. 'I'm asking for your advice here.'

'I was getting to that. He may not be holding back out of respect for you but out of belief,' she told me. 'He's a man of Christian principles. He may not be up for sex.'

'Oh.' This was something else entirely from my own dilemma and a bit of a blow.

Terry's friend, Lilly, who was going to drive two hours to Fredericton tomorrow, to meet up with Terry and me, had had been proud of holding out until her wedding night, I remembered.

Did Butch, a previously-married man, have the same values?

'As to just holding hands, Terry, I don't know.'

'Why don't you talk to him about it?'

'Are you nuts?'

'Talk to him.'

'I couldn't do that.'

3.

'I have something to tell you, Bobbie,' Terry said, as she took off her boots in the apartment hallway.

'Yes?' I imagined she had some further advice for me.

She straightened and removed her jacket. She looked thinner and paler than the last time I saw her. Her golden hair ran down her shoulders in rivulets from an inch of dark near the scalp. But she was smiling. 'I'm done with Don.'

'You mean you're separating?'

'Divorcing,' she said.

'But you said you would stay.'

She shrugged. 'God is shifting and rearranging things in my life.'

I asked her if she was sure. She said she was. Remembering the pressure Veronica had put me under, I left it at that.

Terry had brought Middle Eastern finger food — humus, pitta bread and spicy salad. She laid it out on a cloth on the living room floor.

Mitchel was there. I also got to meet Butch's sweet daughter, Sheena, and her fiancé, who came from Moncton, to stay a few days.

Lilly arrived with a present for Butch and me, a book of devotions for couples she had picked out at the bible bookstore where she worked. I blushed when I unwrapped it.

'Thank you,' I said, handing it to Butch like it was hot.

He did not seem a bit fazed that others already saw us as a couple.

The night before, his mother phoned as I was cooking supper. I liked it when he told her his girlfriend from England was here. But being his 'girlfriend' was not the same as being a couple, which seemed to me something much more rooted, when I was still feeling like a little seedling.

Though I had not ventured all the way up to the threshing floor to muck about — my purpose was marriage — I nevertheless needed pause to try on my new identity.

We all sat on the floor in a circle, exchanging stories, singing Israeli songs and picnicking. It was great fun.

Later that night, at the hotel, Terry, who was staying over with me, confirmed, 'He likes the whole package.'

That was good to hear. 'So do I.'

I was impressed with Butch's total honesty and kindness. He was attentive. He brought me encouragement and laughter. I felt God had a big smile on His face as He watched the two of us.

The only thing preventing me from rushing in headlong was that I did not rush headlong into things.

Terry and I talked into the night, mainly about her desire to go and live in Israel, where, she was convinced that she and I would be involved in some kind of End Times war effort.

Having no church affiliation, she didn't do the basic, sensible thing of referring her visions back to a solid church body. Now that I had the benefit of that type of support through HTB and the pastorate group I'd joined, I was realising that she was something of a maverick, faith-wise.

Nonetheless, I believed many of her words for me were from God. It was her interpretations, the spin she put on them, that I was increasingly having doubts about.

'What about Lonnie?' I asked. His world had been rocked by the breakdown of her marriage.

Her face grew stern. 'Don wants custody. But I've hired a lawyer. He won't get it.'

'Where's Lonnie now?' She had come alone.

'At home. He had school today.'

I frowned. 'How can you say you want to live in Israel and be fighting for custody of Lonnie at the same time?'

Never mind his emotional needs, on a practical level alone, she'd have no right of abode there as a non-Jew. She wouldn't be able to put him in school. She'd have no health cover.

I don't know whether the rambling answer she gave me ever

addressed my question. She finished by saying, 'I think Butch is going to be a vital support person for you for the things to come.'

She meant Israel. She wanted me to live in Israel. It was pretty obvious that the 'mission' was what counted most in her eyes.

Her little boy must be suffering. But there seemed to be no talking to her about this. I made a few further tries at opening a discussion before, saddened for little Lonnie, I let it go.

Being at odds with my friend did not detract from the deep love I had for her.

Later, as I lay in bed, listening to her regular breathing and thinking about Butch, it occurred to me that, with a time delay, the parallels between our lives were continuing.

I saw that the rug might not be the prophetic revelation of a Narnia-type adventure for the two of us, as she believed. It could represent something much more basic, though no less miraculous. What if God had put the rug into Terry's hands to lure me here to New Brunswick, where He could, by happenstance, place me in the field of my Boaz?

What if the story rug told of Terry, heralding me here to lasso my quarry as, below us, her husband galloped out of the picture right and my ex was poised to skin a dead deer before going off to the left?

4.

'She must have been a Christian woman,' I said to Butch. 'Why didn't you want to go?'

He had just shared that, a few months previously, a friend from Smythe Street Cathedral, his home church, where we now sat waiting for Sunday morning service to begin, had invited him on a blind date.

It was a big church. An expectant buzz of conversation surrounded us, above the pop praise coming through the P.A. I scrutinised the assembled congregation. 'Did she attend this church?'

'I don't know.'

'Weren't you curious?'

'I didn't want to go on a blind date and I didn't want to make up a foursome with Garnet and his wife.'

His lack of curiosity was a curiosity to me.

'Mitchel thought I was crazy. *It's been three years*, he said. *That's time enough.*'

'But you didn't listen?'

He draped an arm about my shoulder. I liked the protected feeling and the warm linen smell of his shirt. I tried to catch Terry's eye and share my inner glow. But she was deep in conversation with Mitchel, sitting beyond her on the pew. Beyond him sat Gerry.

'I told Mitchel I wasn't good at choosing women,' Butch continued.

It seemed he'd done most of the child-raising within the marriage and beyond. She had hardly been in touch since the break-up and had taken up with a violent guy who was now in prison.

'Mitchel's answer was, *Your faith is strong, Dad, and yet you don't believe you can ask God for what you want.*

'He got right down on his knees beside the bed. I looked at his mop of red hair and felt he was my reward, I didn't need anything more. A year or so before, he had gotten so messed up by my unstable state that he could hardly read. But now he was tackling the Old Testament, even the hardest bits. We'd worked hard at it as a team, together.'

Mitchel had seemed so mature on our first meeting that it had come as a surprise when Butch had dropped into one of our conversations that he had been through a period of ducking school and hanging out with bad boys, after his parents split.

At this point, one of the pastors, Pastor Wayne, came across to welcome Terry and me to his church. He was excited to learn that I was from London's HTB, a church well-known to him, since he had attended the annual Alpha Conference there, earlier that year.

I had been warmly welcomed by greeters, both at the front entrance and at the door to the sanctuary. For such a lofty, geometric, seventies building, the atmosphere was surprisingly down home and cosy. I decided I really liked Smythe Street Cathedral.

'So?' I prompted, after Pastor Wayne moved on.

'Uh?'

'You were telling me about Mitchel praying.'

A reflective expression crossed Butch's face. 'Sometimes with Mitchel it's like *I'm* the child. I put down the dirty dinner plates I was carrying to the kitchen and got on my knees beside him. He turned to me. "What do you want to ask for, Dad?" I didn't know what could fill the emptiness inside.

'Mitchel seemed to sense my confusion. *Okay*, he said. *Dear Father God, it's time for Dad to stop feeling sorry for himself. It's time for him to live again. Please bring a good woman into his life.* He opened his eyes. *Tell God what you want, Dad.*

'I gave a little cough and said, *Lord, if it is Your will, please send me a good woman who's faithful and loving and strong in faith.*

'*Someone who won't hurt him like he's been hurt in the past,*

Mitchel threw in.

'*Yes, Lord*, I said. *I need for You to pick a good woman for me. And I need You to show me beyond a shadow of a doubt that she is the one.*

'And we both said, *Amen.*'

Wow, he had asked for pretty much the same as I had! Now I knew beyond a shadow of a doubt that we were God-breathed. It was a wonderful feeling.

'Then I remembered something real important,' he went on, his expression sheepish and impish, all at once.

'What was that?'

'I added, *And, if possible, God, could she also be hot?*'

I burst out laughing. 'I asked for fanciable.'

'What's fanciable?'

'Hot.'

It was his turn to laugh. 'Two weeks later, you showed up on my doorstep. I could not believe how fast God worked!'

I felt blessed and highly-favoured to be right where I was, right now.

A countdown to the start of the service had begun on the screens to either side of the raised dais, where choir and instrumentalists were assembling. Behind them was a plain wooden cross, eight or ten feet tall. High above that was a small, stained-glass window that glowed like Jesus' lantern in William Holman Hunt's famous painting, *the Light of the World*.

As Pastor Wayne picked up the mic, I snuggled back against Butch's shoulder. I had prayed for a good man, he had prayed for a good woman and here we were.

Grateful tears welled up.

At this point, I noticed that Gerry's eyes were closed. I nudged Butch and we watched as his slack-jawed head drifted gently onto Mitchel's shoulder.

Terry's face grew perplexed. She looked from us to Mitchel and back again.

'So, who do I get to cuddle up with?' she remonstrated.

5.

The back door slammed as Jamie, no doubt wrapped up warmly, went outside for a smoke.

I was sitting on the couch in the bedroom at Butch's apartment. Through the wall, I could hear Butch talking to Sheena in the kitchen, as he cleared away the supper things.

Mitchel and Jeremy, Sheena's fiancé, were in the living room, watching a programme on t.v. that had a lot of canned laughter. Gerry was in his bedroom at the end of the hall, singing praise songs into his toy microphone.

I said a little prayer: *Father, please give me the strength to broach the subject that's doing my head in. Be with me, guide me in what I should say.*

Butch came in and sat beside me. 'You know, Sheena and Jeremy share a bed every night but they're abstinent. I don't know how they do it.'

I cleared my throat, grateful for what looked like my way in, and trusted because I didn't know what was going to come out of my mouth. 'Can we talk about sex?'

'Sure,' he said evenly, as if I'd suggested we discuss what we had for supper.

'Well,' I begin, my hands working as if I was hoping they'd spin the phrases I needed out of thin air. 'I don't know if you're expecting me to seduce you because there's no way I'd have the confidence to do that. But I have been experiencing... stirrings. So I asked Terry about it and she said you were a man of Christian principles and you might not be up for that.'

'Yes, I am.' Smiling, he put his arm about my shoulder. 'The church doesn't agree with sex outside of marriage.'

'Oh.' That was how it was going to be, then, I supposed.

On the way back to the hotel, we played the Snow Patrol CD I'd brought him from the UK.

When *Chasing Cars*, which I loved, came on, we exchanged glances at one another at the words, Would you lie with me and just forget the world?

Just short of the doors and lights of Reception, he stopped the car in the dark.

'I know you're right for me,' I said. In my head I was thinking, *Spread your cloak over your handmaid, for you are the redeemer.*

He parked up.

'Do you feel bad?' I asked him.

He didn't answer but I knew that he did.

'I don't,' I said. 'This isn't some flash in the pan. This is special and God-led.'

'It's as if we were already married,' he said. 'I already feel as if you're my wife.'

6.

My stay was over, already.

At Fredericton airport, we held hands, eyes on eyes. That was embarrassing and unfamiliar at first but became shared, desired, sought.

'How do you see the future?' Butch asked.

'I don't know,' I answered. 'I think we should try to bring this to a slow boil.'

I was afraid that what we had found might fizz up and fizzle out.

Though he nodded sagely, I was not sure he could do it. The light of hope was there in his eyes.

'I had to pursue you,' I reminded him wryly. 'You let me make all the running.'

'You gave me no sign you were interested.'

'True,' I conceded, 'At first. But then I suggested we could be more than friends and you said, *No*.'

'I didn't say, *No*. I just thought I should wait until I had something to offer you.'

'But I couldn't wait'

'Apparently not.'

We grinned at one another.

'When you said you were coming, I knew beyond a shadow of a doubt that you were the woman God had picked for me.'

'God has blessed us by bringing us together,' I agreed.

'I'll be there soon,' he said. 'I'll get my plane ticket this week.'

He was ready to go racing forward, racing headlong.

We held one another close when they called my flight. He wanted all I was. I wanted everything he was. And we did one another good.

'No secrets,' he said, 'Promise?'

'Promise. Do you promise, too?'

'Yes.'

Alone at Montreal Airport, en route for London Heathrow, I could still feel his parting kiss on my lips.

Chapter 13

1.

The familiar creaks and pops of my house, as I lugged my suitcase through the door, seemed to wipe the week away. I wondered whether that world of pewter lakes and trees and sky had been illusory and the moments of tenderness had happened to somebody else.

I scooped an armful of mail from the floor and carried it to the kitchen. I put the kettle on to make myself a cup of tea and took it to my p.c. where I sat, sipping tea, as it booted up.

Ignoring the unread mail in my Inbox, I wrote:

Arrived home safely. Going to sleep now.

Love

Bobbie

Grrr... Email felt regressive.

2.

'It's the time you waste on someone that counts,' I told Butch, on the phone, later that day.

'It's the time you waste on someone that counts,' he repeated.

I had just shared a bit of the story of Saint Exupery's *Little Prince*. 'The fox is tamed because the Little Prince has allowed the fox the space to find its own courage and inch closer.'

'I like that,' he said.

'Now they'll never forget one another, even though they're apart. And, whenever the fox sees a field of golden corn, he'll be reminded of the Little Prince's golden hair.' I paused to consider what my own memory trigger would be. 'I guess whenever I see countryside through a windscreen of rain streaming down, I'll think of you.'

'Not only then, I hope.'

'No, not only then.'

He laughed. 'Though it sure did rain while you were here.'

Later, he wrote:

Have I tamed you yet? I sure want to.

My reply set him straight:

Seeing as I made all the running, I think it fairer to say I did the taming. And now I've wasted so much time on you, I have no choice but to be committed.

The truth was we had both done the 'taming'. Each, in turn, had stood in an unthreatening way that allowed the other to approach.

As I was thinking about this, the phone rang.

'Hi, Mum.' It was Tania.

Normally, we would chat away about the loves in her life — some guys, mainly horses. Today, however, she seemed subdued.

'You're back.'

'I'm back.' I tried to sound more upbeat than she did, though her gloom was travelling down the line to me.

'How was it?'

'Good.'

'So did you stay with him?' she wanted to know.

'No, I stayed at a hotel.' I wasn't enjoying this phone call. It was like I was the daughter and she was the Mum, asking questions. 'He's coming in January. Maybe you'll be able to meet him.'

'Maybe...'

In actuality, I realised, probably not, since it would be term time and she would be teaching in Birmingham, a good two hours away from home.

'Will Terry come, too?' she asked.

'No, he'll be coming on his own.'

'Ah.'

I took the phone into the kitchen. Rain was lashing the window like a windscreen. The late November afternoon felt like night.

'Are you upset about it, Tania?'

She loved her Dad.

'No, it's good.'

She was trying to sound brave and cheerful, I could tell.

3.

The emails took up again with a vengeance:

To Bobbie:

I keep rerunning sections of your visit here like a favourite movie...

To Butch:

What is between us seems very intense. It could form the basis of a lasting relationship. But we haven't had time to know each other, have we? What we like is the idea of one another. The reality may be different.

To Bobbie:

I like the idea of a future with you. I know you're not ready to commit, commitment takes time. But there's something about feeling loved that's overpowering.

'Why do you laugh when I tell you I love you?' he asked, during the phone call that followed this email.

I couldn't explain, so I ran a little experiment with my eldest son the following Sunday.

'Jeremy.' I was sitting on the couch at his house, watching him iron his shirts for work.

'Yes.' He didn't look up.

'I love you.'

He laughed nervously. A cloud of steam rose from the ironing board.

'Why do you laugh?'

'I don't know,' he said. 'I guess I'm embarrassed.'

'That's how I feel when you say you love me. I'm embarrassed,' I reported back to Butch. I was curled up like a caterpillar on the couch, with a woollen throw over me.

'If it's true, why shouldn't I share my feelings?' he replied.

Flames were dancing in the hearth. It was cosy here in my living room. All that was missing was him. Yet the idea of telling him as much turned my cheeks scarlet.

'I don't know.' I suspected it was a British reserve type of a thing. North Americans had no trouble telling others how much they loved them, I'd discovered. Tania and her friends, the twenty-somethings and below, have caught it. But stoic British oldies like Jeremy, in his mid-thirties, and myself found it tough.

'The words come with a river of heartfelt emotion,' Butch said.

Like Boaz, who praised Ruth for her qualities, Butch praised me and declared his love for me. Though I basked in his words, this was unfamiliar territory. I had never been wooed before. Seth was definitely not the wooing type. He'd made out he was marrying me because I was so keen to get married.

'Don't be afraid,' he said. 'What I say, I mean. I'm very sincere. I won't ever hurt you.'

Our conversations brought us closer and closer. We were in one another's thoughts constantly.

I emailed:

Today, as I took you around with me, I pointed out St. Clements Church which is very pretty, (you know, from the song, 'Oranges and Lemons'?). We walked down towards the Thames where the fairy lights were twinkling on the South Bank. I showed you how to feed your ticket through the machine for the tube and, at Victoria Station, I showed you how to keep going to get through the people criss-crossing in front of you.

To Bobbie:

You've tugged strongly at my heartstrings. I did feel as though I was there.

It's still storming here and not expected to let up until tomorrow. I'm going for a walk at 6 pm. You'd better dress in warm clothing. Don't forget your gloves.

Later, that same night, he wrote:

You were with me every step of the way. I felt such an inner peace. I wish that feeling could remain 24-7. I guess the best way to describe it would be blessed.

The conversations and emails, though beautiful, were mere Band-Aids on an amputation. I missed him and wanted him with me. When I was there, it hadn't felt like a long time until he would visit in January. Now it did.

So much for a slow boil.

4.

Veronica scrutinised me as I stepped into her hallway. 'You look very happy.'

I thought of Naomi, who exclaimed, 'Who are you, daughter?' when Ruth returned, transformed, from her encounter with Boaz at the threshing floor.

'I feel all aglow,' I said, as we hugged.

She led me into the plush living room of her Arts and Crafts home which was like a house beautiful feature in a glossy magazine. We drank tea and chatted.

The burned-down candles of a *Chanukiyah* were guttering on the windowsill, their statement of joy in the Jewish Festival of Light dwarfed by the flashing blaze of Christmas Santas and prancing reindeer going on at the house across the way. Since this was a Jewish household, Veronica had no Christmas decorations. Nor did I. But I was thinking that next year, maybe, I would have some lights and a tree, to celebrate the birth of Jesus.

I told her about my trip to Fredericton. When I had finished, she sighed and laid her hands in her lap. 'Bobbie, even though Seth has behaved like an idiot...'.

My head swivelled in her direction. My eyes widened. Was she finally acknowledging that it was not all my fault?

She was hesitant, picking her words with care. '...the love you've found in this man...'

If I was hoping to be cast in a good light, however, I was about to be disappointed.

'...is not sent by God.'

I bristled. 'And how would you know that?'

'What I mean is you won't be able to remarry, not scripturally.' Her delivery was gentle. Her face was pained. She looked as if she didn't want to have to tell me such things but was compelled, by her beliefs, to do so.

Her voice of conscience made me squirm. It always took me forever to work out whether I was in sin or she was being too narrow.

I thought of the sad stories I was hearing from hurting women at the Divorce & Separation Recovery Course, women who believed that their lives were failures because their marriages had failed, women who thought, because they didn't do bars and nightclubs, that they'd never meet anyone again, women of means who found themselves abruptly counting the pennies, women in their fifties who considered their lives over. These women believed they'd never love again.

I wanted to hearten them.

At the farewell supper for the end of the course the previous week, everyone had looked gooey-eyed at me when, as a facilitator this time around, I stood to announce, 'Last time this course ran, I cringed, like many of you do, about the future and dating. I couldn't imagine there being anyone for me. But, through faith and this course, I've moved on and found the courage to pursue a man. And I'm pleased to report he's now pursuing me back.'

This generated a round of applause.

Veronica was not looking gooey-eyed at me. She had her dogged face on. 'If the grounds for divorce are other than sexual immorality, we are to remain celibate.'

She would have told those women, like she was telling me, that God wanted them to shut up and put up with how things were. He wanted them to suffer. He required them to remain eunuchs.

We revisited my own circumstances. Though the grounds for divorce ended up as mutual consent, Seth had begun dating other women soon after we separated. Giving up on us, he had launched into what was technically adultery. This cut no ice with her.

As I headed back along her driveway at the end of the evening, I reviewed in my mind the points I might have made. I almost turned back to share with her the glib remark Seth had delivered as I left him: 'Marriages come and go.'

But I doubted it would have made any difference to Veronica, so I got in my car and drove away.

5.

My struggle with Veronica was nothing compared to the hard time Tania gave me, a few days later.

'Mummy,' she began, 'Dad's been telling me all this stuff about Butch.'

'*Dad* has?' I was flabbergasted. I hadn't seen or spoken to him in months.

'Yeah, he's been married before,' she said.

She was leaning across the table at me, invading my space, and wearing a determined look that took me back to her babyhood, when she made up her mind to oust one of her brothers and muscle in on a cuddle.

In spite of how annoyed I was that Seth had information I didn't give him, ergo there was behind-the-scenes whispering going on again, I tried to strike a reasonable tone. 'Well, darling, he's fifty.'

'And he's lost all his money?'

'Now, hang on just a moment...' This was too much. 'Where has this come from, Tania?'

I could hazard a guess. Despite Jeremy and Alicia's comments that I looked radiant on my last weekend family visit, they'd passed on reservations about my new relationship. All I'd said was that he went through a hard time financially, after his marriage broke up.

'Has it crossed your mind, Mummy, that this man could be after you for your money?'

She was lecturing me. I was deeply offended. Did she think I was too naïve and ditsy to know what was good for me?

'Are you implying I've nothing else going for me?'

What should have been a lovely evening was rapidly turning to vinegar.

This was my favourite South Kensington restaurant. And the young woman sitting opposite me, Made in Mummy, was so beautiful. Her long, dark hair framed her face and her eyes were the colour of a tropical ocean.

My next remark was below the belt and I knew it. 'What's this sudden interest in what I'm doing, Tania? When your Dad and I split up, you left me to my own devices.'

Things had been very clear-cut to Tania when her parents' marriage ended: I had taken the decision to leave, which had caused her suffering. She wasn't going to offer me any comfort. In her mind, all I had to do to stem my own, self-inflicted pain was reverse my decision.

'That's because he was needy and couldn't cope,' she shot back.

I snorted. He'd never shown me needy and can't cope. 'Your father's been in la-la-land for some years now, I'm afraid. His life is all about him.'

This was clearly not the right thing to say either, but I was furious to have lost my appetite for the costly morsel that I was waving about at the end of my fork.

I took a deep breath, counted to ten and tried again for reasonable. 'Look, Tania, you left me to make my own life and, now I have, you're *being critical and nasty.'*

The waiter approached. 'Tutto bene, signora?'

I stuffed food into my mouth, chewed and forced a smile. 'Very good, thank you.'

Tania leaned forward as soon as he was gone. 'We're all worried for you.'

'*All?*'

A split-screen of talking heads popped into my mind — my family gossiping about my love life.

She set her mouth and shook her head. 'I don't want to meet him!'

'I did wonder about that!'

Tears welled in her eyes. 'I won't ever meet him!'

'I hope you change your mind.'

'I won't!'

She was sounding more like two than twenty-two.

Tania has always voiced opinions that have frustrated me and provoked me to anger. She has also always had the power to melt me. Her present anguish moved me. Despite my own smarting, self-righteous indignation, I wanted to sing her a lullaby by speaking to her lovingly.

The most comforting thing I could find was to encourage her to look the monster in the face and realise it wasn't so very scary.

'I know you're still hoping your Dad and I will get back together,' I told her, 'But, sometime, you're going to have to accept that, though the marriage is broken, I'm not, and neither is your he.'

I don't know how much good it did.

Her parting shot, standing on the pavement at the end of the meal, was, 'I really think you're moving too fast with this.'

She flounced away.

6.

I dawdled back to South Ken tube station. With my family saying, 'beware,' and my friend saying, 'you have no right', I had to consider the possibility that others might be seeing things more clearly than I.

The world had succeeded in ungluing Butch and me a little tonight.

Later, I stood before my computer in my dressing gown, unable to bring myself to write my usual goodnight message to him. Though I had wholeheartedly agreed when he said that good communications were everything, I could not pull off false cheerfulness any more than I could bring myself to set down feelings which, inevitably, would send him directly to the phone.

Exhausted, I clambered into bed and switched off the light, only to toss and turn and switch it on again a few moments later and plump the pillows up behind my back.

'Show me, please,' I prayed.

I turned to my bible, hoping for comforting scripture but it opened at Job 15: *Why does your heart carry you away, and what do your eyes wink at, that you turn your spirit against God, and let such words out of your mouth?*

'I don't understand, Lord,' I said. 'Is this a rebuke for me or for them?'

Perhaps I had spoken out in a way that was displeasing to God. Or was it just that I was Job today, under attack from evil?

'If my relationship with Butch is the right thing, please give me a text that'll give me confidence,' I prayed.

This time, my bible opened at 2 Thessalonians 3: *As for other matters, brothers and sisters, pray for us that the message of the Lord may spread rapidly and be honored, just as it was with you. And pray that we may be delivered from wicked and evil people, for not everyone has faith. But the Lord is faithful, and he will strengthen you and protect you from the evil one. We have confidence in the Lord that you are doing and will continue to do the things we command. May the Lord direct your hearts into God's love and Christ's perseverance.*

I had asked for confidence and been given a text about confidence. I was humbly and tearfully grateful. 'Thank you. Thank you, God. Please direct my heart into Your love and Christ-like patience.'

When I opened my computer the next morning, I found a beautiful picture of a snow angel that Butch had emailed me at just about the time when I would have been arguing with Tania. As I was smiling at it, the phone rang.

It was 4 a.m. where he was. He had not slept for worrying about my silence.

'I thought you might have changed your mind about us.'

'Why?' I challenged, feisty enough, though I was filled with sadness for the pain I had caused. 'Do you think I change like the wind?'

After we discussed all that happened, I realised it would have been better to just share. Hadn't I promised him no secrets?

'It's not surprising, I suppose, that your family feels like this,' he said. 'I don't know how I could ever prove my love for you to those who are telling you to beware of me.'

'What's really sad,' I said, close to tears, 'is that all these people want the best for me.'

'It sure knocks the wind out of your sails, though.'

'Yes.'

'I love you enough to slow things down, if you think that's best.'

'Don't.'

'Are you sure?'

'Derr.'

Chapter 14

'We're in the middle of a big snow storm,' Terry told me.

I knew this already. Butch had told me it was storming when I called him to get the number of where she was. She'd left home for a secret location Don didn't know and hadn't told me.

I supposed it would have been a bit of a cheek to ask her hosts, who were modest church leaders, if she could call England as soon as she took her coat off. However, I wondered how necessary it really was for her to hide from her husband.

And, though she assured me she was keeping in touch with her son, she deflected every question I asked about him. I was concerned that she had left him behind. I couldn't imagine doing something like that.

Though I loved her personality, so vibrant, feisty and fun, I was worried now that something unbalanced was going on. The storm prophecy had been too much for me and I was sad to discover it was still current with her. She was still predicting it and had notified the media, she said. There would be deaths.

Corinne had been having an affair with Don, she maintained. That didn't ring true at all.

And Don had planted bugs in her car to spy on her. That was why she had to escape. He was watching her every move and listening, to discover her secrets.

There was too much innuendo, too many sentences begun and left unfinished. And all, seemingly, to demonstrate to herself and others that she was special and chosen by God.

Her condition would have generated only support from me, had she wanted it. But she pooh-poohed every expression of my fears for her.

She began, yet again, to share visions of Indiana Jones-style adventures in Israel. As her monologue ran on, I stared out of my window at the pale blue, December day. Blackbirds on the lookout for worms were swooping from bare branches onto my back lawn. The

English winter was mild. Where she was, they were hip-deep in snow.

She inhabited a world that was tough beyond my comprehension.

Terry told me that she had spoken to the people in Israel about Butch and me. I think by 'people' she meant Yonaton, who was her usual contact.

So I guessed she'd given him her number.

She sounded a little surprised to report that they were all in favour of the relationship. Their okay seemed to free her to endorse our relationship herself. 'I think he's going to be like a power pack for you,' she said, 'a prayer warrior when you're away from him and a power charger when you're together. I think you'll marry.'

I breathed a sigh of relief, not for the approval from Israel, or hers but because, finally, there was an element of the conversation I could engage in. 'I like that.'

'I don't think it'll take long to get to that. I was told in Jerusalem that this thing is going to be HUGE!'

She was not about to let me forget it.

'When something that huge exists, people need support, loving support.'

She was the one in need of loving support, I thought. It was so distressing. Every good thing that happened to me this year had originated in her. Now she was pushing me away.

Her voice dropped to a whisper. 'You guys have been brought together for the greater good of the mission.'

'What is 'the mission', Terry?' I asked, for the umpteenth time.

In my garden, a juicy worm dangled momentarily from the beak of a lady blackbird before disappearing down her gullet.

'You're going to be ministering to the poor and loving it, Bobbie. I think Butch is going to be a vital support person for you for the things to come.'

I would have been content if my mission amounted to quietly making Butch's life happier.

2.

Near my home, hidden away between a leafy park and a housing estate, was a wending, tree-lined track, lined by an ancient farmhouse and a row of workers' cottages. Here, the birds sang their little hearts out, decibels louder than anywhere else, and the throbbing of cars was absent. It was like a bygone world.

Out for a Christmas walk, alone, I noticed something floating down out of the sky, a yard or so in front of me. I had only to put out a hand for a pure white feather, delicate and pristine, to land in the palm of my leather glove. I wondered what kind of feather it was, goose down, perhaps, or the wing feather of a white dove.

I look up and saw only massed, grey cloud. No bird was in the sky above me. It seemed the feather had fallen from an angel's wing...

Like a Christmas present from God, I took it as a confirmation of His Presence, a 'hi' like the one He had sent me the previous summer, when the wind had lifted to rifle the trees and, just as quickly, was gone.

This time, He had given me something I could keep. I could even include a photo of the feather in my 'Days' montages. (I was counting down the days until Butch came by creating composite pictures in Photoshop of objects and people that were meaningful to us, composed around the number of days remaining until we would be together.)

The feather put me in mind of the start of *Forrest Gump*, a movie that we both liked a lot and had recently discussed. A feather floats down, tugged this way and that by the breeze, and the stage is set for the theme of contrasting the apparent randomness of the world with the individual destinies the characters strive for.

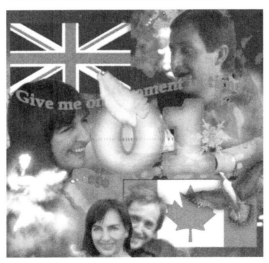

We ended up talking about whether there can be free will when God has a plan for each of us.

'I believe it's our call whether or not we grasp that plan,' I told him. 'Meeting you was an opportunity that might have been lost if I hadn't pursued it. But I was meant to love you.'

'God made us in His image, to love one another,' he replied.

It was the most beautiful thing anyone had ever said to me.

My hand closed over the gift of perfect beauty in my palm. The feather heartened me, for it seemed to confirm: *You're doing okay down there. Keep up the good work.* With all the *opposition surrounding me, that felt very* special.

3.

As soon as I got home, I went to my computer and emailed Butch about the feather:

The physical is very strong for us and I think you feel conflicted about that.

But the way my body feels about you is part of my humanity and God made us in His image and to love one another. The white, fluffy feather confirms everything I feel about how natural that is.

No doubt, I was wrong and Butch was right about the rights and wrongs of sex outside of marriage. The Bible did not condone it.

My comfort lay in Jesus' attitude with the woman caught in adultery. He showed compassion towards her. Nevertheless, having released her from punishment, He instructed her to sin no more.

My difficulty with viewing my behaviour as sin lay in the wonderful blessing of healing that I felt I had received through the relationship He had gifted me with Butch.

Getting ready for bed, I would pause before the bathroom mirror. That breast they cut off when I had the mastectomy then cut off again when the reconstructive surgery failed, the breast that in the end had somehow been cobbled together again, no longer seemed so hideous.

4.

I spent New Year's Eve with Jeremy and Alicia and my granddaughters.

Arriving in the late afternoon, I galloped upstairs to their computer for a rendezvous with Butch and Terry at the Fredericton City Hall webcam.

I have taken to logging on to the city's webcam site, watching the skaters at Officers' Square and the traffic on the Westmorland Street Bridge, always half hoping to be lucky enough to spot his car.

I never was.

Atlantic Canada is four hours behind England. While evening had started to draw in here, it was broad daylight there. Or it would have been, except that Fredericton was in the middle of a snowstorm.

I screwed up my eyes. In front of the ornate City Hall building, two, muffled up individuals were looking up at me. Between the lapses between shots, they jumped up and down and hugged themselves against the cold.

Butch had been quite mysterious about this appointment. I didn't know what to expect.

They were each holding the end of a banner. I leaned in and, through the confetti snowflakes that were falling, read the words: *Happy New Year. I love YOU.*

Wow!

Next thing, Butch was down in the snow, scissoring his arms and legs. He liked sending me snow angels because I wasn't used to the snow and he thought they were cool.

My take on the snow angels was that they were God-inspired. God's sequence of interactions with me had begun with the angels in Terry's camera. So snow angels from Butch seemed part of the continuum, as appropriate as a pure, white feather, falling out of the sky into my palm.

The camera angle did not permit me to see the snow angel Butch drew in the snow for me with his body, but that wasn't the point. The point was the huge honour my shy hero was doing me by braving the stares of passers-by in order to engage with me, on the other side of the Atlantic.

I lay a palm on the screen and whispered, 'I love you.'

'Don't do that, Mum,' Jeremy said, rubber necking around the door. 'You'll leave fingerprints.'

'Come and look at this!'

He came in, tall, dark and handsome, closely followed by Alicia, small, dark and Canadian. She carried a plate of mince pies. As they squinted at the monitor, Butch boomeranged to his feet.

'He's made a snow angel,' I said, 'On the ground, there.'

'You can't see the ground,' Jeremy said drily. His tone implied this was no big deal.

'I can imagine it.'

I hadn't challenged them about what was being whispered behind my back, although, I had started giving a lot of thought to what I shared. I suspected this was fine with Jeremy, who didn't want to hear about his Mum's boyfriend.

Alicia, however, seemed to melt. 'This is something. It's so romantic.'

Jeremy took the plate from her and shoved it under my nose. 'Have a pie.'

Midnight found my little granddaughters tucked up in bed and Jeremy and Alicia yawning on the couch in front of the t.v. Meanwhile, I was sat on the toilet seat cover in the freezing downstairs bathroom, (the only place in the house where I could get a signal on my phone). I had a finger plugging one ear, to drown out Big Ben's solemn chimes on the telly, and my phone clamped over the other.

'I love you so much, Princess,' Butch said. 'Ten more days and I'll be there.'

'I love you, too.' As the t.v. screen exploded into cascades of colourful fireworks, I vowed, 'No more Christmases and New Years like this, apart. Next year we'll be together.'

'And every year after,' he said.

I was expecting to marry him.

5.

Butch's all-too-brief visit to England reinforced that expectation.

Torrential rain as we walked along London's South Bank and in the quaint town of Rye, near the Sussex coast, could not dampen our spirits. We worshipped at HTB and adored the latest show of Canada's *Cirque du Soleil* at the Albert Hall. I introduced him to Indian takeaways, to Valerie and her husband, Matthew, to my brother, Bill, and his wife, Eve.

We had an afternoon in the park with Jeremy, Alicia and the girls. Simon was too far away to visit in Cornwall, as was Tania, in Birmingham.

Inevitably, the joy of being together was succeeded by yet another wrench apart.

Reluctantly, we reverted to our daily round of two-hour phone calls and emails.

To Butch:

God has put us in a position of either/or, rather than and/and. By this I mean there's no way that we can factor the other into our lives as add-ons. When we're together, we pretty much drop everything else and focus on one another. The majority of couples don't do that, at least only when they're on honeymoon — not at the start of things.

I keep reminding myself that's where we are, at the start of things, because it doesn't feel that way. It feels much more established. I think trust underpins that. We trust in the goodness of God's provision and in the other. The honesty makes us behave in ways that could be seen as naive and gullible. It's what makes us like teenagers. It's priceless.

6.

The week before my next trip to Fredericton, Seth showed up unexpectedly on my doorstep. I took him into the living room.

He remained standing. There was little preamble to what he had come to say.

'I've always loved you, Bobbie, perhaps without realising it.' His tone was matter-of-fact. He might have been talking about the laundry.

This was even more unexpected than opening the door and finding him standing there.

'I still do.'

He didn't appear to have put any more thought into his presentation than he had into his delivery. He was wearing his baggy t-shirt and shorts that I had never liked because they swamped his slender frame. His hair was clamped to his head. He must have come here straight from a sweaty tennis match.

What I felt was annoyed.

It struck me that he didn't really want reconciliation. This half-hearted attempt was more of an insult than a compliment. He was flexing his muscles, to see if they still worked, more likely.

No matter what his motivation was, I knew I was done with stoking black memories of the hurts he'd inflicted. They had floated off into the sky when I gave him up to God.

'I'm always unwilling to give my feelings away,' he said. 'I think that's what's been my downfall.'

The phone rang. I jumped.

'Is that...?' he asked.

I was expecting a call from Butch. 'I need to answer this.'

I was as embarrassed as the employee whose boss is in the room when the recruitment agency calls. My cheeks were burning as I lunged past him for the phone.

'I'll go,' he said but moved no further than to sidestep out of my way.

I picked up the receiver. 'Hello.'

I didn't know why my throat felt so dry. I was doing nothing wrong.

'Hi!' Butch's happiness wagged its tail down the phone line at me. 'Just a sec.'

I looked at Seth who nodded and let himself out.

'No secrets, we agreed,' I told Butch. There would be no more trying to avoid passing on stuff he wouldn't want to hear. I took a deep breath and quietly shared that Seth had just gone. I told Butch all he'd said.

There was a long, long silence when I finished.

'If you want to go back with him, I'll back off,' he said, eventually.

'What are you saying? Are you trying to feed me a line that lets me go? Because I don't want to.'

Butch wanted to know whether I'd kissed Seth.

'I don't think you're quite seeing this as it actually happened,' I said and told him the whole episode again.

7.

That night, I dreamt that Butch and I were walking, hand in hand, along a narrow path, beside a cliff edge. Ahead of us, in the distance, was a chapel.

Without warning, he lost his footing. I tried to stop him falling and pull him back up, but I got yanked over the edge, after him. I flailed at the cliff edge, grasped it with my fingertips and managed to cling on. Though he was holding on to my leg, surprisingly, his weight did not drag me down. However, I realised that, sooner or later, my grip would give out and we both would fall.

'Everyone has a moment,' I prayed. 'Is this my moment?' I was asking God if this was my time to die and telling Him I was ready.

What happened next was totally unexpected. Butch clambered up onto the ledge and pulled me up after him!

He saved *me*.

Chapter 15

1.

Everywhere I laid my eyes there was something special — red roses, a heart-shaped box of chocs, little bottles from Body Shop, a leaf-green bathrobe, a mulberry tablecloth, with matching napkins and candles in toning shades of caramel and pink.

'You did so much!' I was overwhelmed by the housekeeping suite Butch had arranged for me.

'I wanted you to be com-for-table,' he said. Com-for-table was his favourite word. 'I rented the room from yesterday so I could get it ready for you.'

This time, I was braving the depths of New Brunswick in the winter. It was February and I would be staying a month.

The night was clear and the stars twinkling overhead as the city hopper aeroplane from Montreal descended towards Fredericton's spires and buildings. I saw the St. John River, petrified, and little puffs of fog rising from the exhaust of each idling vehicle waiting at lights. It was minus thirty something down there.

Nevertheless, I was thrilled to be here.

We drove straight here. He was eager to show me everything he had put in place.

We sat down on the couch, amongst the crimson pillows and soft beige throws he had bought, and I threw my arms around his neck and kissed him.

'I'm closer to you than I've been to anyone,' he said. 'I love you so much.'

'I love you, too. I love you so much.'

We lifted one another's spirits. He saw me as beautiful, sweet and feminine and I became the image he made of me. As for him, he was growing in self-confidence as he basked in being loved.

'Before I met you, my life was just awful,' he said. 'God answered my prayers.'

'And mine.'

'Now life is better than it's ever been.'

'Yes.'

That impish-sheepish grin I was coming to know so well filled his face. 'So...'

He went down on one knee before me and fumbled in his pocket for a little box that he flipped open to reveal a ring. The stone was a deep, dark ruby, fired with scarlet lights. It was flanked by two square-cut diamonds that sparkled like the snow under the streetlight outside.

I choked up. 'It's so beautiful.'

'You're my treasure, Bobbie. Your worth is far above rubies.'

'This is so special.' I had known a proposal was coming. He had asked me what kind of ring I wanted and I had remembered the ruby of the vision I had lying in my sickbed, after my trip to Israel.

Seeing it before me felt as if God was keeping a cryptic promise He had made to me then.

I hadn't anticipated a proposal this trip, let alone tonight, the night of my arrival. I hadn't known that Butch already had the ring.

I took it from its box. The ruby was from Burma, cut in Israel, he said.

'Will you marry me?' He put it on my third finger, left hand.

I clasped his face in my hands and tilted it upwards until our eyes met. 'Yes.'

It was perfect: the two of us so in love, the goodies all around, the cosiness of the nest he had made us, the wonderful, Godly ring, the sweet ask. Perfect.

Our kiss was full of the promise that the blessings we've received would be ours to keep, forever.

2.

We were easy now with silence. The long silences as we drove from 'For Sale' sign to 'For Sale' sign were also a kind of sharing.

After some discussion, we had decided to live in Canada. It came down to the fact that he had an income here and no idea what he might do to earn one in the UK, whereas I could continue drawing down on my private pension anywhere.

I suspected I would soon miss my kids and grandkids. Right now, however, their cold front of disapproval of the choices I was making in my life inclined me to keep out of their way. I had hopes they'd come around in time.

Our search for a home took us past white-capped trees and wedding cake frosted fields. We saw vistas of frozen lakes and rivers, never meeting another vehicle. We were glad to be out here, still close to Fredericton, but far away from the city's blackened ice banks that were taller than me.

Away also from the hubbub of human traffic at Butch's apartment.

Though I trawled the Internet, and so did our realtor, it was Butch who found what looked like a good place, within our budget. The house was not far from a lake and was surrounded by a forest that was criss-crossed by trails to explore on foot in the summer and on snowshoes or cross country skis in the winter, a forest that was full of bear and moose and deer, chipmunks, squirrels and rabbits.

As we got out of the car to view the house, sharp needles of cold pricked my face and tugged at the hairs in my nostrils. Swathed in a cloud of my own steam, I took in my surroundings. I was struck by the tinny silence all around us. Little creaks and cracks gradually began to fill the silence, the discordant percussion of snow.

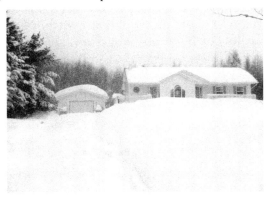

Look at me, in the Canadian countryside, in the middle of the Canadian winter, where I never thought I could manage without a man. And look, here was the man, leading me by the elbow in case I slipped.

We looked around us. Deep drifts masked the front landscaping. We couldn't even hazard a guess as to what it might look like without the snow. Neither could we venture out back to explore the woods that formed part of the 1.4 acre lot.

Inside, the house was spacious and bright, with flowing reception areas and a big, well-equipped kitchen. The master bedroom, at the end of a corridor, had an en-suite. There were four other bedrooms for Mitchel, Jamie, Gerry and guests, and two other bathrooms. There was also a huge detached garage/workshop and a garden shed.

The price tag was similar to the amount my second son, Simon, had recently paid for his two up, two down, Victorian terraced house, three hundred miles from London, in Cornwall. His little house had no garage, no front yard and a tiny courtyard out back.

The realtor suggested I assess the backyard from the dining area patio window.

The expanse of virgin snow, rimmed by fir trees, that I saw sent a thrill through me, for I immediately recognised it as the landscape of my vision that had been the catalyst for my recent picture: She does not Fear the Snow.

I had never imagined that the place of pristine beauty, white and cold, where I looked forward to making some footprints, might really exist. I ached to get out there and stomp about. And, if I sank in up to my midriff, well, Butch would save me.

He came and stood behind me with his arms around my waist. 'So, what do you think?'

I had no misgivings. 'I think God is good,' I said. 'I think this is it.'

By the time the realtor closed the front door behind us, the sky had turned to azure, tinged with crimson. The snow's glow was pinkish under the angled sun. Birds were singing now, not the pretty tweet-tweet of England, but something more melancholic, a song of little, frozen behinds, no doubt.

3.

Tears streamed down all the way to the airport.

This city in winter, flushed with orange under the setting sun, now felt like my reality. I was com-fort-able with the fairy tale that, just a few, short weeks before, my head had struggled to keep up with. It was what I was now returning to that had taken on the quality of a dream.

The realities of this latest trip had helped me get there and not only because we were buying a home. Pastor Wayne, who had been so welcoming at Smythe Street Cathedral, had agreed to marry us, even though we were both divorcees. Butch and I were thrilled, for we were both eager to stand up before God and make our vows.

Had we wanted to wed in my church in the UK, it would have been up to our vicar whether or not to marry us, as divorcees. But we never approached HTB, since Pastor Wayne had already said yes.

We set a date for our wedding, September 6th, the same day as my late parents married in a hurry in 1939, three days after Britain declared war on Germany, the start of World War Two.

As we whizzed past Christmas card clumps of pines and wide lots with grand houses on them, I considered, as I wiped away my tears, that reality was a good place for us to have arrived at. Reality could withstand knocks and offered the security of knowing that a setback was just that, a setback.

When we said our goodbyes, Butch teared up too.

4.

The happy hellos and sad goodbyes were all to do again in April.

Terry came to celebrate a Jewish Passover *seder* meal with us, at our new house. As she stamped the snow off her boots on the porch and came through the door, pretty snowflakes were drifting down outside. It would be my first Passover in a snowstorm.

In her hands was a cardboard box that she left in the hallway.

I was pleased to find she was making a lot more sense and seemed considerably more cheerful than she had been recently. The court had ordered Don to move into his parents' old house, so she could live in their home. She was excited about a trip to Israel she was planning. Butch had lent her the fare for this, since she would be strapped for cash until she received her divorce settlement.

After a short catch-up, she retrieved the cardboard box. Inside was Snowy, one of the kittens that had scratched at the ceiling, the one I had fallen in love with when I visited her, back in September.

She handed him to me. Fluffy and as white as the thick drifts of snow that still lay pristine in our backyard, he snuggled straight into my arms, as if we'd never been apart.

Though all his siblings had found homes, somehow he'd remained. She gave him to Butch and me. I was overjoyed.

Eventually, I needed to move him from my lap and get up to baste the lamb.

Sitting on a chair in what would be our proper dining area, when we got furniture, Terry looked up from her open Bible as I bent over the open oven door. 'I never thought you'd be coming to New Brunswick.' Her tone was wistful. 'I thought I'd be going to Europe.'

What caught my attention was the implied assumption that I was coming here to be near her.

She threw her arms wide. 'You realise that Butch is the only man on earth we could both love and not fight over?'

'This is true,' I laughed. 'The only other man would my brother but he's already married.'

Butch looked up from peeling potatoes. 'Aren't I the lucky one?'

Her face was serious when she told him, 'You have to understand that Bobbie and I will often be away on our travels. Our mission will be taking us to places you've only dreamed of.'

'And I'll stay home and wait for her.' Though his response was delivered light-heatedly, his ironing board shoulders conveyed his resentment.

'I'll find out more in Israel. Why don't you come with me, Bobbie?'

'Sorry,' I said, closing the oven door.

If I were going anywhere, apart from England, it would be with Butch from now on in.

In any case, Simon's fiancé was due to give birth to my new grandchild next month. Sylwia was from Poland and her mother, who ran her own hairdressing business, wouldn't be there. I had promised to go down to Cornwall to support them through the birth.

On top of that, I had a move to Canada to organise.

'This mission of yours,' Butch said to Terry, 'surely it's about saving souls?'

'I guess,' she conceded. Her dark pupils darted across the page of the Bible in her lap.

A potato plopped into the saucepan with a splash.

I concluded that Terry was peeved and Butch was feeling marginalised.

Snowy sauntered through the kitchen, white hair wafting like snow from his tail, held high. Butch liked clean. The hair would drive him crazy. But he loved me and I loved the cat.

I went up to him and gazed into his eyes. 'I'd never be planning to come and live in New Brunswick if it weren't for you.'

5.

This time, when we parted, we knew that the next time I came to Canada would be different. I would be coming for good.

Soon after my return from this trip, I began to dismantle my London life. This sparked yet another vivid dream.

It began in the snowy landscape of my vision/new backyard. A bent, old hag, weighed down by sticks, shuffled towards the woods. From my vantage point, at the patio window, I could see the glimmer of her house lights, flickering between the trees.

I followed her to her snug cottage with its brightly-glowing windows. Deer and squirrels, her friends, gathered around the front door. Inside, I found her relaxing contentedly in an armchair by the fire. She poked socked feet towards it, watching the flames dance. A dog and a cat lay sprawled across the hearth, on either side of her.

The old woman became tiny and entered the fire. I followed. We ran through twisting tunnels of black coals that glowed red and orange. At the very back of the grate, she came to an arched door with metal studs, like that of a mediaeval castle. She opened it and entered a passageway that took her steeply down, down, down, into the darkness. At the bottom, she stood and squinted, unable to make anything out.

Suddenly, a joyful and colourful parade illuminated the black chamber. A Chinese dragon's head danced by, followed by a man in a lion costume. Becoming the old woman, I wondered whether I should join in and, after a moment's hesitation, decided to dance along with them.

Though really quite different in content and context, this dream reminded me of the one I had at Terry's, the dream in which my house was so distressingly bare. Sparked by meeting Butch for the first time, that dream had forced me to recognise how forlorn my love life was.

This present dream seemed also to dwell upon an aspect of barrenness in my life. Though, this time, the house was a cutesy, gingerbread affair, if I wanted more — if I wanted to dance with the colourful parade — I would have to go through fire, heave a heavy door open and stumble about in darkness.

These trials were a metaphor for what I was now going through, prising myself away from everything and everyone I knew, from the things I did and the places I liked to go, from knowing the ground rules and belonging.

Getting permanent residency in Canada could well be an eighteen-month process, I discovered from the Immigration Canada website. I should not even initiate the process until we were married, which was going to be two months after I planned to enter the country, on Canada Day, 1st July, 2008.

Until I got residency, I would have no proper status in Canada. I would be on an extended tourist visa. I would not be allowed to work or have medical cover.

I was used to having the right to live where I lived. In fact, as an E.U. citizen, I could live and work anywhere within the European Union, if I wished to. In the U.K., I could vote and lobby for change. Protection by the law and full National Health Service medical care were my right.

Status was something I had never given much thought to before. I guess I always took it for granted. Now the implications of having none seemed weighty.

With my health history, that gave me a wobbly feeling. I looked for private health cover that would not whisk me back to England if I got sick. If I needed to be hospitalised, I wanted it to be in the same country as my husband.

When I prayed about this, God told me not to worry, I wouldn't get sick. I told Him I'd still like to find the cover, for peace of mind's sake.

The immigration information told me that leaving Canada during the process to become a permanent resident would not be a good idea, as I might not be allowed back in. This seemed harsh. I didn't believe I would be able to stay away from my kids, grandkids and friends for that long, even if some of them were able to visit me in Canada in the interim. I supposed I would just have to take my chances when the time came to plan a trip.

Even though the idea of exchanging my U.K. status for a kind of limbo was upsetting, frightening even, I forged ahead with dismantling my life.

I offered my U.K. home for rent and had to endure prospective tenants picking holes in it. My colour scheme was yucky, my garden too small, I didn't have an eat-in kitchen, the apartment block at the end of the road looked potentially dodgy...

I was hurt. I thought my house and its location were great.

I arranged to ship my furniture to Canada. Scanning the Canadian Customs documentation supplied by the shippers, I realised that none of the categories of duty-free importer matched me. I wasn't a landed immigrant or a returning resident. I wasn't importing wedding gifts. The shipping company warned that a false declaration would be penalised: the onus was on me to get it right.

My days grew as long as the to-do lists I was writing myself and I was in danger of going under, of morphing back into Mrs. Angry again.

6.

My phone conversations, morning and night, with Butch sustained me, especially when he talked to me of our home. He spoke of rabbits on the front lawn, of birdsong and blue crocuses.

One morning, as he sat on the porch steps talking to me, a rabbit came right up to him.

'Like those deer Terry and I met?' I teased.

For someone of such deep faith, he was a terrible sceptic when it came to signs and wonders, especially his sister's.

'No,' he whispered. 'It's right here, at my feet.'

The story he told next seemed to confirm a shift in his thinking. 'The other day, Mitchel reminded me of one of Terry's prophecies that

I can't explain away. Just before I met you, she said I wouldn't be renewing my contract on the apartment. She saw us happy like never before, living in a beautiful house, with trees around it, like this one.'

'Wow! What did you say to that?' I asked.

'I said, *There's only one way out of this apartment and that's through hard saving. It'll take years.*'

'And how long has it taken?'

'About eight months.'

We both laughed.

God's ways were lovely. I imagined His knowing smirks as He brought Butch vicariously to Israel with us, first through Butch's prayer, tucked in the Western Wall alongside Terry's 'I'm Your girl', then at King of Kings, as she dedicated the angel photos she didn't know she was snapping to him.

Butch initially thought those were of her golden hair, flopped in front of the lens.

'By the way,' I asked, 'what was on the note you had Terry slip into the Western Wall?'

'It was a prayer for God to bless my family, I think.'

'It was answered,' I said.

'Yes, it was,' Butch said. 'He's blessed us all.'

God had no doubt enjoyed a further little snigger of foreknowledge as a raven dropped Butch's sandal out of the sky onto his chest, causing him to jump up. This was not only a subliminal message to Butch to get moving. It brought him once again into the realm of supernatural synchronicity Terry and I were experiencing, in this instance through our bird encounters.

'Perhaps the rabbit really has something it wants to tell me,' Butch said, after I reminded him of the shoe-toting raven.

His laughter was like warm rain on my tense shoulders. He loved it there, at our house. I knew I would, too.

7.

My run-in with Simon took place on a Tuesday evening, early in May.

He and Sylwia were planning to get married, soon after the birth of their baby. The late May date they had tentatively set for this hinged on their baby's arrival. He was already a few days overdue.

It coincided with Butch's next visit to England. Naturally, I wanted to bring him to the wedding.

Simon had other ideas. He phoned to let me know that Butch was not 'one of us' and would not be welcome.

Disheartened, I tried to change his mind. 'If Tania wanted to bring a guy, any guy, to your wedding, he would be welcome.'

I sensed his discomfort but he was determined. 'Dad will be there.'

I had already considered that I would appreciate a heads up if Seth ever intended to bring a girlfriend to an event I was attending. I felt I owed Seth the same courtesy. Though I was reluctant to call him after our last meeting, I had already done so.

When I asked him whether the presence of my fiancé at Simon's wedding would make him uncomfortable, he'd told me no.

'He was okay with it,' I said.

'But I'm not,' Simon said.

With a sigh, I realised my son was making me choose between his wedding and spending time with Butch during his forthcoming visit. I refused to allow my family to dishonour my fiancé in this way.

Irate and with heavy heart, I said, 'I won't be coming, if Butch isn't welcome.'

And there the matter was left.

I planned to try and talk him round when I went down there for the baby's birth.

8.

Tania had hardly sat down to lunch in my dining room the following Saturday, before she began picking an argument. 'How can you be so selfish as to leave us behind?'

She was home for the weekend. Her year of teacher's training was almost completed.

'I'm not leaving anyone in the lurch,' I retorted. I didn't need this. My nerves were already frayed from the strain of planning my departure. 'I wish you had the faith, trust and support for me that I've always shown you.'

She leaned forward, ardent, wearing her school teacher face. 'You're not putting your family and their needs first.'

I slouched back in my chair, thinking dark thoughts. This wasn't fair. Wasn't I allowed to seek happiness?

'What needs?' I said. 'Everyone's fine.'

Jeremy and Alicia were happy together. They were fantastic parents to my granddaughters.

Simon and Sylwia were expecting their first baby.

Tania, who was planning to move back to teach locally next year, still had her bedroom in the former marital home, where her Dad still lived. She was staying with him now, as she usually did. She had a huge circle of friends and a dizzy social life.

'We think you should get a pre-nup,' she said.

My eyebrows shot up. My eyes narrowed. I wondered where this North American-sounding term had sprung from. *'We?'*

'Yes, all of us.'

'I'm not even going to ask who you mean.'

Clearly, my three children had closed ranks and were advancing on me with bayonets attached.

She explained why she thought I needed a pre-nuptial contract: it would be sensible to safeguard my assets from my husband, whom she assumed to be a run-around and a gold-digger. When she was done with her character assassination, I thrust my ruby ring under her nose.

'You've not even noticed this.'

'Did *you* pay for it?' she sniped.

'If you're going to be this nasty, we won't be able to hang out,' I shot back. There was a lump in my throat. My eyes were prickling. 'Why can't you just be happy for me?'

'Because you're being way too hasty, Mum,' she said demurely.

9.

I lay in bed that night, tossing and turning, feeling battered.

That afternoon, during my weekly visit to Jeremy's family, he'd grouched: *Why do you have to marry this person, anyway? Couldn't you just live with him?*

I was shocked at such words from my son, who set the institution of marriage and the family on a pedestal.

I told him as calmly as I could, given that anger was churning up my insides, that I had no desire to live in sin. Why would he expect me to do that when I wanted to confirm my commitment to the man I loved?

It had been a tough week with all three of my children.

Veronica, too, was still heaping negativity on me. In the end, I gave her an ultimatum: if she couldn't wish me well in my marriage, then she couldn't be my friend. She said she'd pray about the situation.

The life they would all have me lead was the life of the evening I had just spent: cooking and clearing away, taking a bath, reading, watching t.v., going to bed, alone.

Perhaps I might have been more tactful and forced things to move more slowly, for their sakes. Even as I considered this, however, I knew I couldn't have done it. I had been too miserable for too long.

When God is blessing you and you know it, you don't hold back.

The wind was gusting hard outside. Somewhere a burglar alarm was ringing, on and on.

What popped into my mind, as I prayed about this situation, was Snowy.

The thing I'd noticed about Snowy, as the new kid on the block, was that he would look on, totally unperturbed, while Yoshi, Butch's scaredy cat, went into hissy fits over his presence on her territory.

'Dear God,' I prayed, 'Until my family come around, please grant me the patience and perseverance of Snowy. Let me stand apart from all the things they say and do. And please allow me to receive some comfort from your Word.'

I found Ezekiel 14:22 and 23:

Yet there will be some survivors—sons and daughters who will be brought out of it. They will come to you, and when you see their conduct and their actions, you will be consoled regarding the disaster I have brought on Jerusalem—every disaster I have brought on it. You will be consoled when you see their conduct and their actions, for you will know that I have done nothing in it without cause, declares the Sovereign LORD.

This passage was indeed a great comfort to me for it promised that things wouldn't always be as bad as they were now.

10.

'We'd like you to stay and have an ultrasound,' the nurse said.

My heart jumped. 'Did something show up on my mammogram?'

This was only supposed to be an annual check-up. I had come alone.

'It's procedure, just something we want to look at and make sure of. It may be nothing at all.' She wore a fixed, Stepford Wives' smile. 'The radiographer can see you in about ten minutes.'

I looked to a woman patient sitting opposite for a reaction of some kind — a sympathetic smile would have been welcome. But her nose was firmly in her magazine.

'Calcification.' My voice sounded like it belonged to someone else. 'I've been told before that I probably have calcification... in the good breast.'

It was the only one under discussion. The rebuilt breast had an implant that couldn't be compressed for a mammogram.

'The ultrasound will give us a better picture,' the nurse said. 'Please wait here.'

The seats were covered in blue vinyl. The walls were lavender, the floor mottled grey lino. In showing off its hygiene, the atmosphere of this brand new hospital was one of cold detachment.

'I have to feed my meter,' I called back as I strode away. The nurse stared after me. 'I'll be right back.'

Amazingly, the world outside was still running as normal. It was a blousy, late spring day. The car park was a good few minutes' walk from the main entrance. As I walked, birdsong came in surround sound from the foliage. The fledglings up in the trees were new life. I was old, perhaps obsolete.

By the time I fed coins into the pay machine and took my ticket, I was shaking. As I leaned across the driver's seat of my car to replace the old one, I realised I needed to sit. I sat in the driver's seat. The key was in my hand. The temptation was there to drive away, pretend this wasn't happening...

There had been four of us, friends together, during my cancer treatment. Vivienne, from synagogue, who was already my friend before we got sick, died a few years back, aged fifty eight. Vicky, who I got to know at group counselling at the Cancer Help Centre, died the year before her, aged forty-four. I met Sally at the same time I met Vicky. Two years ago, she found out she had a recurrence. She has refused all treatment and has stopped going for check-ups.

Of the four of us, I was the only one who, so far, had remained well. I had just turned fifty-six.

I looked from the key to the ignition and knew that I could not live like Sally, on a knife edge.

I texted Butch: *If you can, please call my mobile. X*

It rang within seconds.

'Hello, Princess.' His voice was warm. 'How are you?'

I tried to sound breezy. 'Oh, a bit flustered. I've got a call back on my mammogram. They want to do an ultrasound.'

He sounded concerned. 'Are you worried?'

'No. I don't think there's anything wrong, really. Well, I don't feel like there's any... Maybe a little.'

Suddenly, all our lovely plans seemed to be hanging in the balance, the house we wanted to live in together, our wedding, even. I'd thought nothing could stop us. But this could.

'Are you all right?' he asked.

'Bit stunned.'

'I'm here.'

He was funny. 'You're three thousand miles away!'

'No, I'm here.'

I take a deep breath and found I was able to be practical. 'Look, they're expecting me back. I'll contact you after.'

'Straight after, okay?'

'You would come, wouldn't you, if I was sick?'

'Yes,' he said. 'I'd be there right away. But I'm sure...'

'And, if...'— I was getting out of the car now — 'If I was really sick, you'd stay?'

'Of course I'd stay.'

I walked back through the rows of cars with my phone held to my ear, talking to Canada.

'I'd have to stay here for treatment. I wouldn't qualify for medical cover over there, you see.' I took another deep breath. 'If it came to it, you'd stay with me until the end?'

'But, Bobbie...'

'Would you?'

'Yes, I would.'

I knew he meant it. He had held the dying in his arms in the special care homes he had owned and managed.

'Thank you, Butch. Thank you.' I had reached the main entrance. A sign said no mobile phones were allowed. 'I have to ring off.'

'Just a sec', Bobbie. *Heavenly Father, please help and support my fiancé, Bobbie, today as she faces these tests. Please allow them to show no trace of anything wrong. Grant her perfect health. And, please, if it should be that anything is wrong, then heal her now, I ask, before the ultrasound. Let it show totally clear. I pray this in Jesus' Precious Name and thank You. Amen.*'

'*Amen,*' I echoed.

I went back in far calmer than I had come out.

Three quarters of an hour later, I called him back from the car park.

'All clear!' I jumped up and down. 'She couldn't find a thing, Butch, I'm clear!'

Chapter 16

1.

I had to raise my voice above the strains of lively Israeli music travelling down the phone line. 'Terry, have you contacted any of the people whose names I gave you?'

'Everyone's away from Jerusalem right now. It's Independence Day.'

'You've spoken to no one from King of Kings' English-speaking congregation?'

I had looked up the names of the leaders for her online but she obstinately refused to refer any of our story back to any kind of authority.

The music got suddenly much louder.

'Someone's having a party!' she cried. 'They're dancing the *horah* in the street below my room.'

It sounded like they were having a good time.

'Just a sec. I'll close the window.'

The sounds become muffled.

'How about the rabbi who prophesied over your angel pictures, have you seen him?' I asked, frustrated that she was such a maverick.

'Yonaton was attacked!' she said. He was the one she had stayed in close touch with in the fourteen months since her meeting with the rabbi. 'He was ambushed by ultra-Orthodox Jews as he delivered food packages to the poor in Galilee.'

Sadly, I knew that these things happened to Messianic Jews in Israel. Jewish believers in Christ were reviled by other Jews in Israel. 'I'm very sorry for that.'

'He lost six teeth! He looks terrible.'

I was sure Yonaton was a good man. My problem was that Terry had passed on so many of his words and visions about 'the mission' and my role in it that I didn't know what to think anymore.

Abruptly, she changed tack. 'I have some really important news, Bobbie! There's a second rug!'

'Really?'

'I had to pick it out. It was in the warehouse behind the store...'

'Which store?'

'The Messianic Jews'.'

'Yonaton's friends?'

'Yes, Bobbie.' My interruptions made her tetchy. '*We have another rug for you*, they said, *if you can pick it out*. And I did, Bobbie, I did!'

Here was another lavish gift of a rug. Suspicion resurfaced. I wondered whether these people had an angle and I wondered that such considerations didn't seem to concern her at all.

'All the rugs in the back were rolled or piled up,' she went on. 'I looked through them and said, *Is this the one?* They cried, *Yes, sister!* and started praising God and rejoicing. With all those rugs, gee, it was a miracle I picked the right one!'

She was very engaging. I felt a tingle of excitement, in spite of myself.

'This one's much bigger than the first one. It's beautiful. It's a wedding rug...'

'A wedding rug?'

And I was getting married...

'I've taken some pictures. I'll email them to you when I get back,' she said.

'You're still on to be Butch's Best "Man"?'

We had asked her when she visited us in April.

'Of course. What should I wear?'

'Pants?'

We both laughed.

She lowered her voice confidentially. 'I've learned a lot more about the mission... but I can't share it with you over the phone.'

This was an approach I had come to know well. She liked to keep me dangling.

'Everything in God's good time,' I replied, not letting her.

2.

I had little time to dwell on the things going on in Terry's life. I had a move to Canada to organise. Before the packers came to take my furniture away, goodbyes needed to be said. I was short of time and didn't want to hold two parties. I invited all my girlfriends, Jewish and Christian, to a bring-and-share farewell supper.

'So, how does everybody know Bobbie?' someone piped up as soon as everyone was seated.

My heart sank. Now my secret would come out: although the

Christians knew I was Jewish, the Jews didn't know I was Christian.

I supposed I must have half envisaged this when I organised one gathering. I hadn't thought it would happen quite so overtly, however, going around from person to person, with half of them saying they knew me from synagogue and the other half from church.

As we went around the room, I could see the cogs turning in my Jewish friends' minds. One of my Christian friends even worked at HTB as an administrator for the Alpha Course.

To my amazement and relief, my Jewish friends did not sniff at me, snub me or get up and leave. Curious to find out more about the similarities and the differences, they asked my Christian friends all about their beliefs and practices.

This was unexpected. My preconceptions had been totally awry. I was dumbfounded.

One Jewish friend spoke of the Jewish-Christian-Muslim friendship organisation she was involved in. I never knew.

The conversation was lively, the atmosphere friendly. The questions that came my way displayed a genuine desire to know what had brought me to where I was.

I should have found the courage to share long ago, I realised. I should have trusted the relationships, rather than get stuck on the labels.

But having such great friends made the prospect of leaving even more bittersweet.

3.

Terry visited Butch soon after her return from Israel. She took the wedding rug she brought home with her and had him take pictures of it to send to me. I was amazed. Many aspects of it spoke powerfully to me.

Unlike the hunting rug, which was in reds and yellows, this rug was predominantly blues and greens. It told a pastoral story of peasant life, a child growing to manhood and leaving his father and mother to cleave to a wife. The story unfolded over three scenes.

At the top, the hero was a baby, nursed by his mother, who sat with other women as they worked at domestic tasks. Grown to a young man in the rug's middle image, he relaxed with his parents, who were now older. At the bottom, he was a shepherd, facing his bride, who stood across a stream of water from him, with a pitcher in each hand.

If the two were to become one flesh, one of them had to cross that strip of water, which was my situation. If the bottom scene illustrated where I was headed, the top, with its women at their domestic tasks around a nursing mother, showed what I was leaving behind. After helping to deliver little Solly the previous month, I had stayed on to cook and keep house for my son and daughter-in-law while she got used to motherhood.

The youth of the middle scene played the flute, a little apart from his mother and father, as they sat, facing one another. This made me think of Mitchel, who was just finishing Grade 11 at school.

I didn't want him to feel that he no longer belonged, like this youth appeared to. I wanted very much for us to become family. But he was almost grown up and it would take a lot more than just moving in for that to happen.

We had made a good start, however. Mutual respect and liking had been established. I was confident I could be a solid rock for him and help nurture him along his chosen path.

The mother of the lad on the rug sat at the very centre of the whole tableau, spinning yarn. I liked to think that she also span the family's story, turning the strands of their life into fine thread. She was old, in her twilight years. I hoped she reflected my destiny, my happy ending.

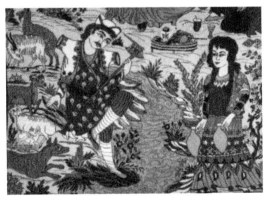

I saw this new rug as confirmation that I had found the purpose I set out to seek in Israel, some eighteen months before. I was at once the bride of the bottom image, the mother's support of the top and the spinner of stories at the centre.

The skills on my resumé, my business sense and creativity, were the ones I tended to talk about but the wedding rug opened my eyes to what I did best of all. It was subtle, so subtle that I had never really stopped to consider it. I was a great homemaker.

Homemaking was something I always did in the in-between times.

Perhaps that was why I never noticed it too much. I worked, I volunteered, I raised children: these were projects. Homemaking was more fluid. It consisted of this touch and that touch in my home décor, of bringing fresh flowers into the home and watering indoor plants, of cooking tasty meals, welcoming visitors with teas and coffees and cookies, keeping up to date with the washing and ironing so that clothes were ready to be worn when wanted, plumping up pillows and putting out fresh towels.

God knew what purpose would truly fulfil me and was giving it to me. He was making me complete.

I wanted to ask Terry what made her pick this rug but, when I tried to call, she didn't answer her phone. When I thought about it, I realised she hadn't emailed me since she got back, either.

4.

Butch came for a fleeting visit just before my home was returned pretty much to how it looked before my furniture went in it. I would be left with nothing more than a rickety garden table and chairs and the spare bed, after everything was packed into a container and shipped off to Fredericton, NB, via Halifax, Nova Scotia, several weeks ahead of my departure.

The idea was that it would arrive only a short while after I got to Canada.

The burning issue of whether or not I would bring Butch to Simon and Sylwia's wedding had been resolved ahead of this visit.

The issue became irrelevant. There were two reasons for this.

Firstly, when Butch went to book his ticket, he decided to come to England a week before he originally planned. This was because the fares of the airline that flew direct from Fredericton to London during the summer were considerably cheaper, the earlier in May you flew.

Secondly, little Solly was born a full thirteen days after Sylwia's due date. I went down to Cornwall the day before she was to be induced but she went into spontaneous labour almost as soon as I arrived. I was honoured when Sylwia invited me into the delivery room to help deliver my grandson.

It was a long haul for poor Sylwia. However, the result was a gorgeous little boy, with masses of dark hair and liquid, brown eyes.

I got lots of cuddle time with him when I stayed and helped keep house while Sylwia recovered.

Because he arrived so late, the date of the wedding was put back to June.

When Butch came to England, we drove down to Cornwall. It was a lovely part of the country at a lovely time of year. We enjoyed long coastal walks and strolls around Cornish gardens.

We were in Simon and Sylwia's area. They had not previously met Butch. I was delighted they said they wanted to meet him. We all got on great together.

5.

My days after Butch left continued full to bursting. Ready or not, I was flying out of here on 1st July.

The phone rang one morning as I was erasing the records of my life with a £10 shredder, one sheet at a time. Butch was drinking his first coffee of the day, sitting out on our front porch with green grass and trees and birds singing all around him.

I had been up since 4.30 am, when the dawn chorus became deafeningly raucous in the back bedroom, making further sleep impossible.

His voice was dreamy as he described last night's moon. 'It sat heavy in the sky like a big yellow balloon, filled with water. I can gaze for hours at moons like that.'

I couldn't wait to be gazing at moons with him. I took a breath and tried to leech some of his calm from him. Then I told him about another strange dream I'd had.

'We were in one of those New York traffic tunnels I've seen on the disaster movies,' I said. 'We came to a border. I was worried that the customs officer might decide not to let me pass but our lovely baby, who was placid and easy, charmed him.'

'We had a baby? I'd love to have a baby with you.'

I didn't want to go there. The years we had been denied together would be too obvious, the admission that we had found one another too late to produce children too painful. So I made a kind of a joke. 'Unless we turn out to be Abraham and Sara, that's unlikely. The baby stood for something else, our love, maybe.'

'But you feel like you're in a dark tunnel, do you, princess?'

'I do right now. The customs officer needed a cheque. You printed it out, ready for me to sign, and the officer let us through. I sat down, close to the barrier, to breastfeed. But the feeding took a long time, the night was coming and we'd hardly gone any distance. I wondered if there was some way to speed things up, like taking a plane.'

'I guess everything you have to get done is getting you down?' he suggested.

'Everything I'm doing involves taking things apart. It's soul-destroying.'

Soon after we hung up, my mobile phone peeped. He'd sent me a text: *Just smile, I'm holding your hand. I'll help you through your day, every step of the way. Xoxoxo*

6.

A couple of weeks before I was due to leave, the phone rang early one morning.

'Terry's disappeared!' Butch announced.

'Disappeared?'

His voice sounded strained. It was still night where he was. 'She hadn't been to the house in more than a week, so Don used his key and went inside.'

She had been living in their home, Don just across the yard in his parents' former home.

I saw scenarios of big rows ending in violence, Don furious with the court's decision to let Terry live in the log cabin he built, while he was demoted to the little, old house.

I saw my friend's poor, broken body languishing in some forgotten gully, for the wolves and coyotes to feast on.

'Everything was packed up, like she was moving out,' he went on.

Ah, that put a different complexion on things. I couldn't see him waiting to vent his passion while she packed everything away first.

'Perhaps she's with friends again,' I suggested, remembering how she'd used the homestead of a couple of religious leaders as a hideaway from Don, the previous winter.

'Don's already called everyone he can think of. No one's seen or heard of her. He says the kid's upset.'

I was very sorry to hear this. Even though I wasn't fully up to date with the custody situation regarding Lonnie, a surge of anger went through me. My understanding was that they were dividing the time with him between the two of them. If that was correct, she'd now reneged on that arrangement, without even preparing her son first.

I couldn't begin to imagine how awful he must be feeling.

'Why would Terry abandon her own son?'

It didn't make sense. She had retained a lawyer to fight for custody.

'Terry wouldn't just strike out completely on her own,' I continued. 'She'll contact us soon.'

He sounded doubtful. 'Only if she wants to.'

His remark concerned me. As her brother, he knew her better than I did.

'What about the wedding? She was looking forward to being your best man.'

'That's still two and a half months away,' he said. 'There's plenty of time for her to show up again.'

I hoped so. We were supposed to be galloping towards one another, about to become sisters.

The idea of running away was so alien to me that I had a hard time understanding why she would take such a course of action. My failure to comprehend took me back to worrying about her safety. This was less painful than thinking that she didn't trust us enough to allow us the opportunity of helping her with the challenges she was facing.

'How can she just drop us?' My irritation masked a niggling sense of guilt that I had somehow failed to take proper care of my friend, again.

'Perhaps she's just gone off the rails,' Butch said.

'Like the storm thing?'

I peered through the bedroom blind at the morning sun, splashing paint across the sky, and heaved a sigh.

I had a lot on my mind. Nothing in this move had been simple but I had found a tenant who seemed reliable and a buyer for my car. I had also found health coverage that would allow me to stay in Canada, and receive treatment there, should I fall sick.

Guilt or no guilt, I was way too busy right now to go chasing after Terry, if she didn't want to be found.

7.

I was sitting on the stairs, with my lunch perched on my knees, when a text message arrived from Tania:

Are you never going to call me?

I'd love to hear from you, I texted back.

Why aren't you there for me?

I've stuck up for you and put you first your whole life.

There's been 6 weeks of silence.

Not so, check your email inbox.

I had emailed her snippets of my news, as usual. She hadn't replied.

The landline rang. It was her. We talked about her job.

She called again later. I was eating my supper this time and watching a pair of squirrels through the bannisters. They were chasing one another's tails, on the patio outside.

'I want to talk,' she said.

I decided to make it clear straight off that I wouldn't hear another bad word about Butch. 'No more bad-mouthing my fiancé, no more trying to run my life.'

'Okay.'

She thought it was her turn. 'This is what I want...'

I couldn't allow this. Her will, mingled with my own desire to please her, were a potential recipe for torment. She had treated me disrespectfully. I thought she should talk to me differently.

'I'm the Mum,' I interrupted. 'I'm in charge here.'

She took that, too.

I asked her if she would come to my wedding.

'Of course.'

The directness of her answer surprised me as much as the fact that it was a yes.

This was wonderful news. I tried my luck further. 'Will you be my bridesmaid?'

I expected a refusal but, again, came an enthusiastic, 'Yes!'

'That's great!'

She scheduled a surprise — mother and daughter time — at the weekend.

My laughter, after I rang off, almost tipped over into tears.

8.

When we got to the train station at the start of my mystery mother and daughter day, my dearest friends stepped out from the shadows behind the ticket office.

Tania had planned a great day out for us all that included lunch, a massage and a mini-facial at a spa in a landmark South Bank building. We spent large chunks of our day drinking cappuccinos in the café overlooking the Thames and reminiscing on times past spent together.

At the end of the afternoon, when we moved on to a bar near the London Eye, Alicia joined us. I was very pleased that she'd made this effort.

Then, much to my surprise, Veronica walked in. The two of us hadn't spoken since I told her of my wedding plans. She had left my house, unable to congratulate me, but here she was to wish me God bless, even though drinking sangrias in a fashion bar was hardly her kind of thing.

Well done, Tania!

There were tears when Valerie dropped us home that evening. Tania got out of the car and went indoors. I sat on a little, talking to Valerie.

'See you in September, as they say,' she finished up, sounding emotional.

(She and her husband were coming to the wedding.)

'Yeah, thanks.'

I got out of the car and took a step towards my front door. But I turned back. 'I love you, Vally Pally.'

She got out and hugged me. 'I love you, Bobbie.'

Such an admission of mutual affection was a big deal for a couple of reserved Brits.

I stood on the pavement with tears in my eyes and watched her drive away. I would miss her.

'Thank you,' I told Tania, inside. 'That was a wonderful day out.'

'Hen party,' she corrected.

'Or bridal shower.'

'You're turning into an American.'

'Canadian, maybe.' I grinned at her. 'I shall never forget it.'

'You're very welcome,' she said, grinning back.

Tears pooled in her beautiful turquoise eyes. I took her in my arms.

'One thing, Mum.' Her tone was serious.

'What?'

'Promise me.'

'Promise you what, sweetheart?'

'Promise me you wouldn't be too proud to come home, if it all went pear-shaped.'

'I'm the Mum,' I said, defensively.

'No, Mum, you have to promise me this.'

'Okay. I promise.'

She still didn't believe I knew what I was doing.

Chapter 17

1.

When my plane landed in Halifax, Nova Scotia, my passport was stamped with a six-month tourist visa, just like any other visitor who hadn't abandoned her whole life to be here.

Waiting for my connecting flight, I felt very differently from on previous visits. I was still excited to see Butch, but I felt dejected and totally dislocated, at the same time. Being in a different country from Solly and my granddaughters, Shoshi and Tali, was going to be the hardest thing of all.

God turned this difficult day around for me. The heavenly show He put on as I flew on to Fredericton, brought a big smile to my face.

Looking glass lakes far below reflected the blue skies that stretched into infinity. As we passed over the Bay of Fundy into New Brunswick, snow-white cloud angels lined up to greet me. They leaned in towards my porthole, flapping pink and ginger-streaked wings and blowing wafting trumpets, to mark my arrival.

Later, as Butch and I strolled, hand-in-hand, through Fredericton's pretty downtown area, a pure white feather, identical to the one that had floated out of the sky into my hand last Christmas, drifted down in front of my eyes. All I had to do was put out my hand to catch it.

Even Butch was impressed. 'Do you think it came from one of the angels that welcomed you?'

'They were clouds, Butch,' I said drily. 'They didn't have real feathers.'

I beamed at him. The truth was I was delighted at his new-found openness to the idea that God could and did communicate with us.

'Real special anyways, eh?'

My fingers closed around this further sign of God's approbation 'Definitely.'

2.

We spent those summer evenings lying out on the lawn in front of our house, Butch, Mitchel and me, dreaming dreams and seeing visions, as we counted the stars above us and the fireflies that glowed amongst the tree trunks all around.

Our days were filled with turning the house into a home and wedding arrangements.

Pastor Wayne asked me if I would like to be baptised ahead of the wedding. I was eager to be baptised. If someone had offered me baptism before now, I would probably have accepted but nobody had.

My baptism in front of the whole congregation at Smythe Street Cathedral, my new home church, officially confirmed the new creation I had become and bonded me to that church for all time.

I always found Sunday morning worship there moving. I was filled to brimming with gratitude for the abundant blessings God had showered upon me.

The big, plain, wooden cross feat the back of the dais featured in a vision I received several times over. I saw, and felt, a heavy headdress on my head, pulling me towards the cross by elastic strands like stretched chewing gum.

I was puzzled by this vision for some time. Eventually, I was led to a reference to the helmet of salvation in the Book of Ephesians, Chapter 6. In this, the apostle Paul invited his readers to don a metaphoric suit of armour and pray in the Spirit with all kinds of prayers and requests, including that it might be given to him to speak boldly to others about the gospel of the cross.

I felt honoured and happy to have been given a helmet of salvation. Receiving it fostered in me a strong desire to speak boldly about my faith and write my story.

That story was a Ruth story. Like her, I came into the Land of Israel destitute, where I was moved to declare my faith. Like her, I received the blessing from God of a new husband.

The three locations where my story unfolded were like beloved daughters, each with her own personality. It began in Israel, with her sultry beauty and Middle Eastern volatility. It was consolidated in serene England, so secure in her identity. It would finish in spirited Canada, wild and free. It was inconceivable to me that any one of the three might be out of my life for good.

Hand in hand with Butch, I could live happily in any one of them. Why, I might even brave Israel…

3.

September 6th was soon here.

When my parents married in 1939, there had been no time to

organise a bridal gown for my mother. My dress was modelled on a sepia photo I had of the printed frock she wore. I had long treasured this photo. Mum looked very beautiful and very happy.

The dress had puffed sleeves and a swaying, Ginger Rogers skirt. The fabric I chose was white chiffon, with hints of rose and saffron. Copying the dress brought my mother to our wedding.

She would have loved Butch.

A dressmaker from my former synagogue made my dress. It was too precious to risk letting it travel in the hold, so I carried it, folded in a plastic bag, inside my rucksack, when I flew to Canada.

My beautiful bridesmaids were Tania and Butch's daughter, Sheena, whose own wedding was barely a month away. Sheena and her future husband hoped one day to have special needs residents of their own.

They wore ivory, knee-length dresses and strappy shoes. With their hair done in up-dos, they both looked gorgeous. We all carried red, pink and cream roses, the colours Butch and I had chosen for our 'romantic' wedding theme.

Terry did not come. She had phoned a week before the wedding. She told us she had been in Israel. This tallied with what Lilly, who we invited to the wedding, had told me, namely that Terry was flying in and out of Israel and staying in northern New Brunswick, in between times.

I had no idea what she was doing in either location. She talked for just long enough to give the impression that she probably wouldn't be at our wedding, although she never did say this outright.

I was sad my friend seemed to have dropped me when I had just moved to a place where I hardly knew anybody. I thought she might be at a low ebb and too proud to let me see it. I kept her in my prayers. As she had struck out on her own, I prayed for her safety. And I prayed that she should find some stability.

Butch thought she probably just didn't want to see their mother.

We made my son, Simon, best man instead. He did a great job with his best man's speech, which poked fun at his mother, rather than at the groom. It was wonderful to have him there.

Mitchel and his elder brother, Michael, were our ushers.

My brother, Bill and Eve, his wife, flew in from England. Bill was to give me away. Valerie and her husband also came. Butch's sister, Norma, and her husband travelled up from their home in Boston, Mass.

We would have liked to have little Lonnie at the wedding but fetching him would have involved an all-day round trip and we already had a houseful of international guests to look after.

I was late getting to the church. Though I realise brides are generally late to their own weddings, in my case, it was not intentional. All began well. The stretch limo we hired from Moncton, sixty miles away, arrived at the house on time. But, as my brother, my bridesmaids and I got in, the chauffeur said, 'Christchurch, right?'

'Yeah, right,' I said. Christchurch was the Victorian Cathedral downtown. He was teasing with me.

But no. He really didn't know where we were going to, neither did he know his way to Smythe Street Cathedral or, for that matter, around Fredericton at all. Since none of the rest of us did either, he drove around, looking for it.

As we crossed a bridge at the wrong end of town, I became rattled that only the word Cathedral had reached my chauffeur, when we had clearly told the limo company that Smythe Street Cathedral was our destination.

By this time, I might have been excused for going into a panic. There was a distinct possibility I might miss my own wedding.

I didn't. I prayed and gave it up to God.

I later learned that Pastor Wayne, trying to reassure Butch, who was clock-watching, said, 'Don't start to worry unless it gets to 2.15.'

He must have started pacing the floor, for it was 2.23 when we finally poured out of the limo. The wedding was supposed to be at 2. Our pianist began to play 'Flying without Wings'. First Sheena, then Tania, processed up the aisle to the podium. When I finally entered on Bill's arm, poor Butch almost ran to grab me and bring me up to join Simon, Sheena, Tania and Pastor Wayne on the platform.

We had chosen Psalm 1 for the groom's reading, which was read by Butch's mother. Its message was that the man who delights in God's law will, like the tree planted by streams of water, yield much fruit.

The reading for the bride came from Proverbs 31 and was read by Bill: *Who can find a virtuous wife, for her worth is far above rubies? The heart of her husband safely trusts her, so he will have no lack of gain. She does him good and not evil all the days of her life...*

I looked deep into Butch's grey-green eyes and read the wave of emotion there as we stood, hands linked, before Smythe Street Cathedral's huge, wooden cross. Secure in our salvation and in one another, we spoke tender verses from Song of Songs:

This is my beloved and this is my friend.

Set me as a seal upon your heart, as a seal upon your arm, for love is as strong as death, jealousy as cruel as the grave.

My dove my perfect one is the only one.
My beloved is mine and I am his.
I am my beloved's and my beloved is mine

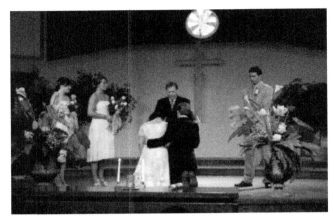

As we spoke these words, I felt rising inside of me the liquid love that God sends down through the Holy Spirit, in exactly the way I experienced it, without realising what it was, that first time at King of Kings in Jerusalem. There, God took me, a despairing Naomi, who thought her happiness all behind her, and began a work of transformation into a Ruth bride.

At HTB, in London, he showed me the forgiveness of the Father and accepted me into His Kingdom.

Here, at Smythe Street Cathedral, in Canada, he was making me a disciple, ready to work for that Kingdom in whatever capacity pleased Him.

I had a beloved church in each of my beloved countries.

After Pastor Wayne married us, we got into the stretch limo as man and wife, and returned home, with Butch directing the chauffeur.

The weather was fine for the reception and we were glad of the shelter an open-sided tent provided. The sunshine was nothing short of a miracle. Earlier that day, almost as soon as Butch and Mitchel left for the church, I faced a real dilemma. The Weather Channel began flashing red hurricane warnings at me.

'Should we set up in the garage?' the caterers wanted to know, as soon as they arrived. The garage, freshly painted, was our Plan B, in case of bad weather.

There was no one else to ask but God. I prayed a little prayer and, since I had no twinge of misgivings when I was done, answered them confidently, 'No, on the lawn.'

And that was where we had our refreshments, followed by a New Brunswick feast that included salmon and dill dip, local chicken, local fiddleheads and blueberries.

Our mutual sons, Simon and Michael swung one another as a merry fiddler struck up a reel. Gerry showed off by dancing a jig. The fiddler serenaded us through our wedding waltz and entertained us through our meal.

We finished the afternoon with a blissful white chocolate and raspberry wedding cheesecake and champagne. I stood to share with our guests the amazing journey that had brought me here.

I spoke of the vision I had had of snow and pine trees. 'I took it to symbolise a fresh start in life,' I told them. 'I had no idea that pure white landscape was my actual destination. I cannot say with any honesty that I do not fear the snow — I have seen how the winters can be here — but I enjoy making footprints.'

At this point, much to the horror of Butch, who saw what was going on but did not want to interrupt my speech, Gerry knocked back his champagne like lemonade.

To the best of our knowledge, Gerry had never consumed alcohol before in his life. He was quite the showman sober and would be bound to make a display of himself tipsy. Also Butch, as his caregiver could get into real trouble with the Province of New Brunswick, who paid him to look after Gerry, if his Downs Syndrome charge wound up drunk.

Unawares, I carried on. 'I thank God for putting Butch and me together. He is the man I prayed for, someone who is kind, a believer and also fanciable.'

Though everyone smiled, some of the North Americans looked bemused.

'Hot. She means hot!' someone clarified.

I wound up with, 'I'd like to invite you to join us in toasting our union.'

As Gerry raised a second glass, Butch lunged forward to take it from him. However what he had already consumed was enough to cause him to play the clown even more than usual for a while. Then, like the Dormouse at the Mad Hatter's Tea Party, he laid his head on the table and went to sleep.

In the evening, we went for a walk around the subdivision. Anyone who felt like coming tagged along. As we walked, the sky grew menacing. As we rounded the final corner home, a roaring wind began to shake the trees.

Heavy droplets of rain burst like bombs on our heads. Butch and I sprinted, hand in hand and laughing, for the shelter of our house. The others were hard on our heels.

Now it began. Here came the hurricane.

Butch's Testimony

In 2007, I was going through quite possibly one of the lowest times in my life. Extreme marital problems had led to divorce and I had walked away from a very successful business. All this left me broken and confused. I was not the strong, confident person or father that I had been in the past but managed to raise my son, Mitchel, on my own.

Day after day, my son was watching me sink deeper and deeper emotionally. This was beginning to scare him, I think.

After watching a movie about God on television, he began to read his Bible and seek a relationship with God. Sunday after Sunday, he would ask me if I would go to church with him. I thought that going to church would mean that I'd have to quit smoking and commit to something I wasn't ready for. I found just living a struggle.

But Mitchel persevered and, one day, I had to say 'yes' to my son and take him to church. We decided we would try Smythe Street Cathedral. I remember the Sunday we went, I think I brushed my teeth at least three times, along with mouth wash and anything else I could find to mask the smell of cigarette smoke. I realize now that God wanted me there just as I was.

When I was young, I accepted the Lord but was not a faithful follower and really thought that in order to be a Christian, I had to be perfect. I was not able to be perfect so I lived life the way I wanted to. I can say that even though I was far away from God my whole life, He was always there for me.

I've been shown favour, time and time again.

My first visit to church was comforting in a way. I enjoyed the praise music and was warmly greeted by Pastor Wayne and others but really couldn't wait to get home.

My son was very happy that we had gone to church. I soon felt God speaking to me and my son and I began to read the Bible and pray together.

Life seemed so much better. I was excited to go to church and really felt as though life was headed in the right direction. The Lord started blessing my life immediately with a new job that I liked and was comfortable in.

I thought I would never be interested in another relationship or a date with a woman, but there seemed to be a bit of desire, after more than three years of being completely alone.

I spoke to Mitchel about this. We decided that maybe if we prayed that the Lord would choose the right woman for me. I asked the Lord: 'If it's Your will for me to have a lady, I would like You to put her in my life. I would like her to be a Christian and hot, if possible.'

I had nothing to lose by asking.

Two weeks later, a woman came knocking on my door with my sister. To make a long story short, she is now my wife.

The Lord has always looked out for me. I've failed him, over and over, but He has always been faithful to me.

Butch Cole

About the Author

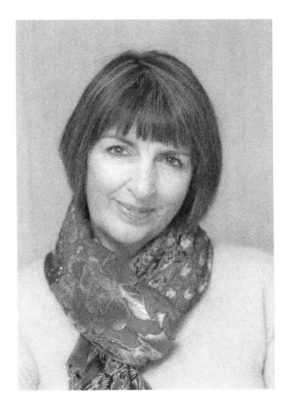

Bobbie Ann Cole is a writer, speaker and teacher of creative writing, specialising in personal memoir and testimony and bringing Bible stories to life.

She lives with husband, Butch, in an 1840s home in Fredericton, New Brunswick, Canada, and a 2012 home in Canterbury, England, both of which she loves.

She enjoys three children and three grandchildren in England and three step-children and step-grandchildren in Canada.

Read the sequel

Love Triangles
Discovering Jesus the Jew in Today's Israel

www.love-triangles.com

A Jewish woman's unconventional quest to find Jesus in modern Israel

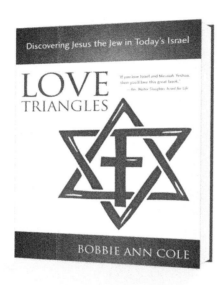

"Moving and well written, Bobbie Ann Cole's story of making Aliyah to Israel with her husband, Butch, combines history, Scripture with accounts of Messianic Jews and Christians living there from around the world. With open, heartfelt honesty, Cole shares vital insights on the courage and determination that Messianic believers require to sustain their calling in Israel."
— *Ben Volman, Chosen People Ministries*

"Bobbie has captured what matters. This book is not about theological principals; it's about love."
— *Adrian Glasspole, British Messianic Jewish Alliance*

"A vibrant, captivating read that effectively interweaves Israel's ancient and modern history with biblical references and the author's own personal experiences. Sparkling with intelligence and peppered with sage observations, Love Triangles is a fearless and thought-provoking labor of love born out of Cole's deep passion for both the Messiah and the country of Israel."

> — *Sally Meadows, award nominated singer/songwriter, author "Beneath That Star"*

"Her love of the Land of Israel and the Scriptures shine out as the author narrates her Aliyah journey."

> —*Judith Galblum Pex, author "Walk the Land"*

Discover:
- How Jesus used Jewish festivals to underscore His message.
- The story of Jesus' Bar Mitzvah.
- Why Jewish atheists may move to Israel but not believer Jews.
- Why Judaism rejects Jesus as Messiah.

A Gift for You

THE ISRAEL JESUS LOVED

Get closer to Jesus and His homeland with this FREE Ebook

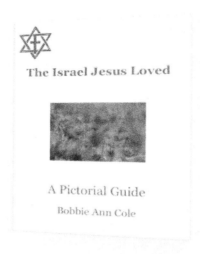

The Israel Jesus Loved

A Pictorial Guide

Bobbie Ann Cole

jesus-ebook.com

Printed in Great Britain
by Amazon

58305545R00122